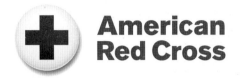

# American Red Cross
# First Aid/CPR/AED

**Participant's Manual**

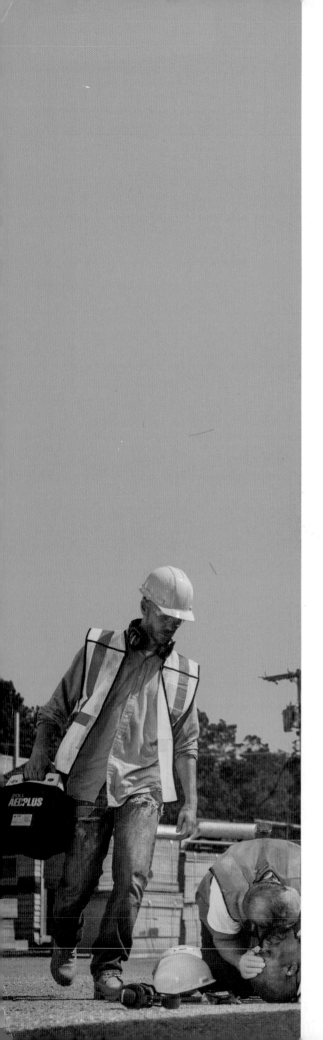

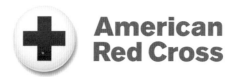

## American Red Cross

This participant's manual is part of the American Red Cross First Aid/ CPR/AED program. Visit redcross.org to learn more about this program.

Published by StayWell

Printed in the United States of America

ISBN: 978-1-58480-665-3

# Acknowledgments

The *American Red Cross First Aid/CPR/AED Participant's Manual* was developed through the dedication of both employees and volunteers. Their commitment to excellence made this manual possible.

# Dedication

This manual is dedicated to the thousands of employees and volunteers of the American Red Cross who contribute their time and talent to supporting and teaching life-saving skills worldwide, and to the thousands of course participants who have decided to be prepared to take action when an emergency strikes.

# Table of Contents

## PART 1
## FIRST AID BASICS / 1

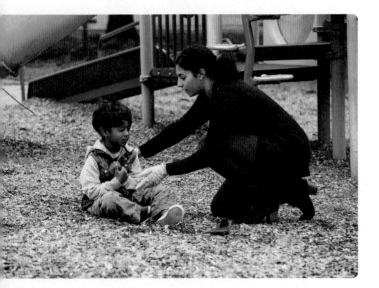

## PART 2
## FIRST AID FOR CARDIAC EMERGENCIES AND CHOKING / 34

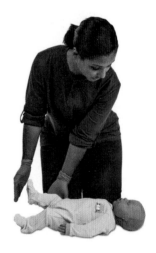

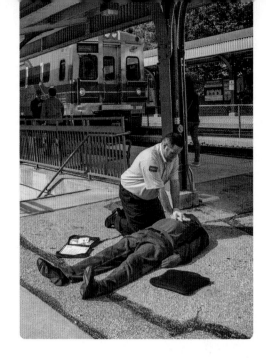

# PART 3
## FIRST AID FOR COMMON ILLNESSES AND INJURIES / 74

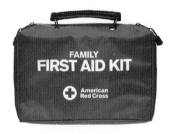

# APPENDICES

# PART 1

## First Aid Basics

# 1

# BEFORE GIVING CARE

**B**eing knowledgeable and skilled in providing first aid can help you to make your workplace, home and community a safer place to be. When a person is injured or becomes suddenly ill, your quick action can prevent the injury or illness from worsening, and it may even save the person's life. Although every emergency situation is unique, understanding basic principles of giving first aid care will always serve you well.

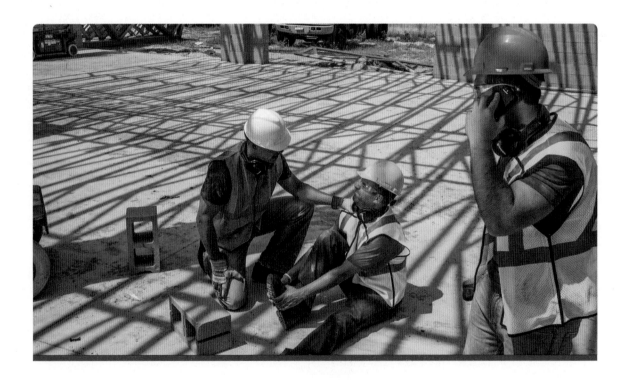

# Preparing for Emergencies

By definition, emergencies are unexpected situations that require immediate action. But by expecting the unexpected and taking general steps to prepare, you can increase the likelihood of a positive outcome should an emergency situation arise.

By reading this manual and participating in an American Red Cross First Aid/CPR/AED course, you have taken an important first step in preparing for emergencies. You will learn the concepts and skills you need to recognize emergency situations and respond appropriately until advanced medical personnel arrive and take over. Once you have learned these concepts and skills, review and practice them regularly so that if you ever have to use them, you will be well prepared and have the confidence to respond.

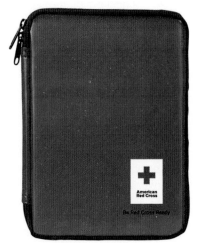

Make sure you have ready access to items that will make it easier to respond to an emergency, should one occur. Keep a first aid kit in your home and vehicle (Box 1-1), and know the location of the first aid kit and automated external defibrillator (AED) in your workplace. Download the American Red Cross First Aid app to your mobile device so that you always have a first aid reference at your fingertips.

## Box 1-1. **First Aid Kits**

You can purchase first aid kits and supplies from the Red Cross store (redcross.org) or a local store. Whether you buy a first aid kit or assemble one yourself, make sure it has all of the items you may need. Check the kit regularly and replace any used or expired supplies. The Red Cross recommends that first aid kits include the following at a minimum:

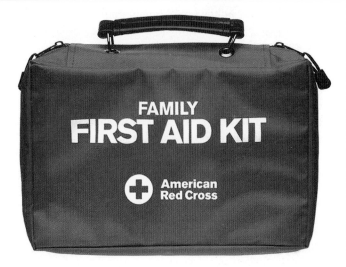

- 2 pairs of latex-free gloves

- Latex-free adhesive bandages (3 of each of the following sizes):
    - 1 × 3 inches
    - ¾ × 3 inches
    - Large fingertip
    - Knuckle

- 8 sterile gauze pads (2 × 2 inches)

- 8 sterile gauze pads (4 × 4 inches)

- 1 roll of adhesive cloth tape (2½ yards × ⅜ inch)

- 4 roller bandages (2 inches or 3 inches × 4 yards)

- 4 roller bandages (4 inches × 4 yards)

- 1 elastic bandage (3 inches or 4 inches × 5 yards)

- 3 or 4 triangular bandages (40 inches × 40 inches × 56 inches)

- 1 36" malleable radiolucent splint

- 1 unit antibiotic ointment, cream or wound gel

- 4 sealable plastic bags (1 quart) or 2 chemical cold packs

- 5 antiseptic wipe packets

*(Continued)*

Box 1-1. continued

- 2 hydrocortisone ointment packets (approximately 1 gram each)

- 2 packets of chewable aspirin (81 mg each)

- 1 space blanket

- 1 CPR breathing barrier (with one-way valve)

- 1 pair of utility shears or scissors

- Oral thermometer (nonmercury/nonglass)

- Tweezers

- First aid manual

For a list of the recommended contents for a workplace first aid kit, see ANSI/ISEA Z308.1-2015—*American National Standard for Minimum Requirements for Workplace First Aid Kits and Supplies.*

Keep a current list of emergency telephone numbers in your mobile phone, by the telephones in your home and workplace, and in your first aid kit. Most communities are served by the emergency telephone number 9-1-1. If your community does not operate on a 9-1-1 system, look up the numbers for the police department, fire department and emergency medical services (EMS) system. Also include the number for the national Poison Help hotline (1-800-222-1222) on your list. Teach everyone in your home how and when to use these numbers.

Take steps to make it easier for EMS personnel and others to help you should an emergency occur:

- Make sure your house or apartment number is large, easy to read and well lit at night. Numerals are easier to read than spelled-out numbers.

- Keep relevant medical information, such as a list of the medications that each family member takes, in an accessible place (for example, on the refrigerator door and in your wallet or mobile phone).

- If you have a chronic medical condition such as diabetes, epilepsy or allergies, consider wearing a medical identification tag to alert responders to the presence of the condition in case you are not able to. You can also create a digital medical identification tag in your mobile phone that can be accessed without unlocking the phone (Figure 1-1). In addition to information about chronic medical conditions, blood type and so on, you can enter contact information for the person you would want contacted on your behalf in case of an emergency.

In a life-threatening emergency, every second counts. By preparing for emergencies, you can help ensure that care begins as soon as possible—for yourself, a family member, a co-worker or a member of your community.

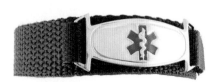

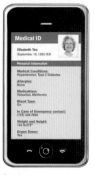

A                    B

**Figure 1-1.** A medical identification tag (A) or an application on your phone (B) can give responders important information about you in case you are not able to.

# Understanding Your Role in the EMS System

The **emergency medical services (EMS) system** is a network of professionals linked together to provide the best care for people in all types of emergencies (Box 1-2). As a member of the community, you play a major role in helping the EMS system to work effectively. Your role in the EMS system includes four basic steps:

1.  Recognizing that an emergency exists.

2.  Deciding to take action.

3.  Activating the EMS system.

4.  Giving care until EMS personnel take over.

## Recognizing that an Emergency Exists

Sometimes it will be obvious that an emergency exists—for example, a scream or cry for help, a noxious or unusual odor, or the sight of someone bleeding severely or lying motionless on the ground are all clear indications that immediate action is needed. But other times, the signs of an emergency may be more subtle, such as a slight change in a person's normal appearance or behavior, or an unusual silence. Your eyes, ears, nose and even your gut instincts can alert you that an emergency situation exists (Box 1-3).

## Deciding to Take Action

Once you recognize an emergency situation, you must decide to take action. In an emergency, deciding to act is not always as simple as it sounds. Some people are slow to act in an emergency because they panic, are not exactly sure what to do or think someone else will take action. But in an emergency situation, your decision to take action could make the difference between life and death for the person who needs help.

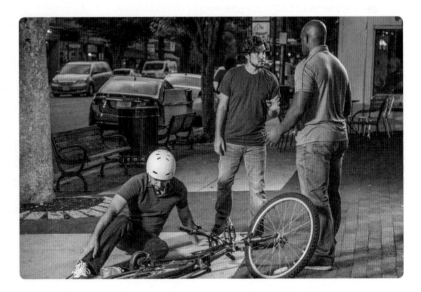

Your decision to act in an emergency should be guided by your own values and by your knowledge of the risks that may be present. However, even if you decide not to give care, you should at least call 9-1-1 or the designated emergency number to get emergency medical help to the scene.

# Box 1-2. The Emergency Medical Services (EMS) System

The EMS system is a network of professionals linked together to provide the best care for people in all emergencies.

The system begins when someone sees an emergency and decides to take action by calling 9-1-1 or the designated emergency number.

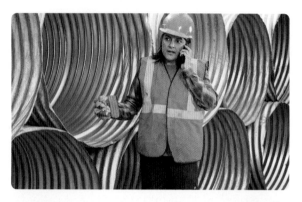

This action allows the EMS dispatcher to take down information about the emergency and provide it to the trained EMS professionals who will respond to the scene. Many EMS dispatchers are also trained to provide first aid and CPR instructions over the phone to assist the lay responder until the professional responders arrive.

EMS professionals have advanced training that allows them to provide medical care outside of the hospital setting. EMS professionals have different roles and responsibilities, based on their level of training:

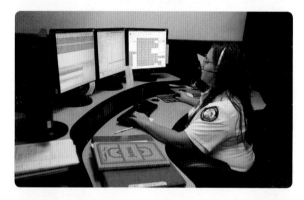

- Emergency medical responders (EMRs), such as police officers, fire fighters, ski patrol personnel, park rangers and athletic trainers, are trained in some of the most time-sensitive lifesaving measures, such as using an AED or an epinephrine auto injector. (Unlike lay responders, EMRs have a legal duty to act in an emergency.)

- Emergency medical technicians (EMTs) are qualified to provide more comprehensive basic life support care at the scene of an emergency, in addition to performing the duties of an EMR.

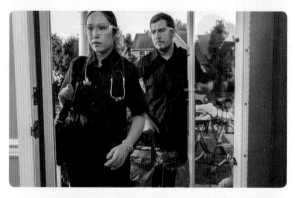

- Advanced EMTs (AEMTs) are EMTs who have received additional training that qualifies them to perform certain advanced life support skills and administer some medications at the scene of an emergency.

- Paramedics are trained to give the highest level of advanced medical care at the scene of an emergency, including the administration of medications and advanced airway support.

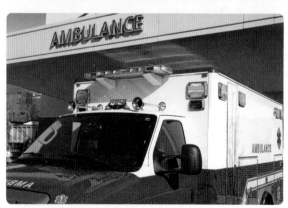

Once on the scene, these professionals will take over the care of the person, including transportation to a hospital or other facility for the best medical care if needed.

# Box 1-3. **Signs of an Emergency**

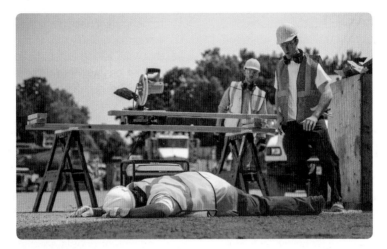

## Unusual Sounds

- Screaming, moaning, yelling or calls for help
- Sudden, loud noises such as breaking glass, crashing metal or screeching tires
- A change in the sound made by machinery or equipment
- Unusual silence

## Unusual Sights

- A stopped vehicle on the roadside or a car that has run off of the road
- Downed electrical wires
- Sparks, smoke or fire
- A person who suddenly collapses or is lying motionless
- Signs or symptoms of illness or injury, such as profuse sweating for no apparent reason or an uncharacteristic skin color

## Unusual Odors

- A foul or unusually strong chemical odor
- The smell of smoke
- The smell of gas
- An unrecognizable odor
- An inappropriate odor (e.g., a sickly sweet odor on a person's breath)

## Unusual Behaviors

- Confusion in a person who is normally alert
- Unusual drowsiness
- Personality or mood changes (e.g., agitation in a person who is normally calm, irritability in a person who is normally pleasant)

Many different fears and concerns can cause a person to hesitate to respond in an emergency. Understanding these fears and concerns can help you to overcome them:

- **Being uncertain that an emergency actually exists.** Sometimes people hesitate to take action because they are not sure that the situation is a real emergency and do not want to waste the time of the EMS personnel. If you are not sure what to do, err on the side of caution and call 9-1-1 or the designated emergency number.

- **Being afraid of giving the wrong care or inadvertently causing the person more harm.** Getting trained in first aid can give you the confidence, knowledge and skills you need to respond appropriately to an emergency. If you are not sure what to do, call 9-1-1 or the designated emergency number and follow the EMS dispatcher's instructions. The worst thing to do is nothing.

- **Assuming that the situation is already under control.** Although there may be a crowd of people around the injured or ill person, it is possible that no one has taken action. If no one is giving care or directing the actions of bystanders, you can take the lead. If someone else is already giving care, confirm that someone has called 9-1-1 or the designated emergency number and ask how you can be of help.

- **Squeamishness related to unpleasant sights, sounds or smells.** Many people feel faint or nauseated when confronted with upsetting sights, sounds or smells, such as blood, vomit or a traumatic injury. You may have to turn away for a moment and take a few deep breaths to regain your composure before you can give care. If you still are unable to give care, you can volunteer to help in other ways, such as by calling 9-1-1 or the designated emergency number and bringing necessary equipment and supplies to the scene.

- **Fear of catching a disease.** In today's world, the fear of contracting a communicable disease while giving care to another person is a real one. However, although it is possible for diseases to be transmitted in a first aid situation, it is extremely unlikely that you will catch a disease this way. Taking additional precautions, such as putting on latex-free disposable gloves and using a CPR breathing barrier, can reduce your risk even further.

- **Fear of being sued.** Sometimes people hesitate to get involved because they are worried about liability. In fact, lawsuits against **lay responders** (nonprofessionals who give care in an emergency situation) are highly unusual and rarely successful. The majority of states and the District of Columbia have **Good Samaritan laws** that protect people against claims of negligence when they give emergency care in good faith without accepting anything in return (Box 1-4).

## Box 1-4. Good Samaritan Laws

Good Samaritan laws, which protect the responder from financial liability, were developed to encourage people to help others in emergency situations. They assume a responder will do his or her best to save a life or prevent further injury. Good Samaritan laws require the responder to use common sense and a reasonable level of skill and to give only the type of emergency care for which he or she is trained. Good Samaritan laws usually protect responders who act the way a "reasonable and prudent person" would act if that person were in the same situation. For example, a reasonable and prudent person would:

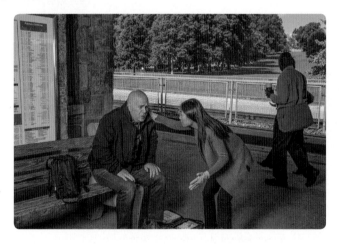

- Move a person only if the person's life were in danger.

- Ask a responsive person (or the parent or guardian of a minor) for permission to help (consent) before giving care.

- Check the person for life-threatening conditions before giving further care.

- Call 9-1-1 or the designated emergency number.

- Continue to give care until more highly trained personnel take over.

If a lay responder's actions were grossly negligent or reckless, or if the responder abandoned the person after starting care, Good Samaritan laws may not protect the responder. For more information about your state's Good Samaritan laws, conduct an Internet search or contact a legal professional.

# Activating the EMS System

In a life-threatening emergency, activating the EMS system is an important thing for you to do.

Activating the EMS system (Box 1-5) will send emergency medical help on its way as fast as possible. The sooner emergency personnel arrive, the better the chance for a positive outcome. At times you may be unsure if advanced medical personnel are needed. You will have to use your best judgment—based on the situation, your assessment of the injured or ill person, and information gained from this course and other training you may have received—to make the decision to call. When in doubt, make the call.

---

## Box 1-5. **When to Activate the EMS System**

Call 9-1-1 or the designated emergency number for any of the following emergency situations and conditions.

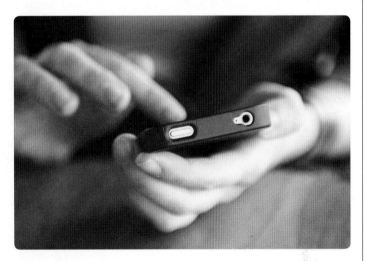

### Emergency Situations

- An injured or ill person who needs medical attention and cannot be moved
- Fire or explosion
- Downed electrical wires
- Swiftly moving or rapidly rising flood waters
- Drowning
- Presence of poisonous gas
- Serious motor-vehicle collision

### Emergency Conditions

- Unresponsiveness or an altered level of consciousness (LOC), such as drowsiness or confusion
- Breathing problems (trouble breathing or no breathing)
- Chest pain, discomfort or pressure lasting more than a few minutes that goes away and comes back or that radiates to the shoulder, arm, neck, jaw, stomach or back
- Persistent abdominal pain or pressure

- Severe external bleeding (bleeding that spurts or gushes steadily from a wound)
- Vomiting blood or passing blood
- Severe (critical) burns
- Suspected poisoning that appears to be life threatening
- Seizures
- Signs or symptoms of stroke (e.g., drooping of the face on one side; sudden weakness on one side of the body; sudden slurred speech or difficulty speaking; or a sudden, severe headache)
- Suspected or obvious injuries to the head, neck or spine
- Suspected or obvious broken bone

Most people in the United States call 9-1-1 for help in emergencies. But in some areas of the United States and in many workplaces, you many need to dial a designated emergency number instead. If you live or work in an area where 9-1-1 is *not* the number you should call in an emergency, make sure you know what the designated emergency number is.

Phone carriers are required to connect 9-1-1 calls made from a mobile phone, even if the phone does not have an active service plan. In most areas, you cannot text 9-1-1. You must call! Unless you have confirmed that the 9-1-1 call center in your area supports texting, you should always call.

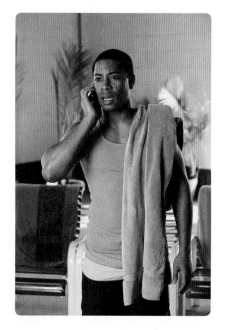

## Giving Care Until EMS Personnel Take Over

First aid care can be the difference between life and death. Often it makes the difference between complete recovery and permanent disability. This manual and the American Red Cross First Aid/ CPR/AED courses provide you with the confidence, knowledge and skills you need to give care to a person in an emergency medical situation. In general, you should give the appropriate care to an injured or ill person until:

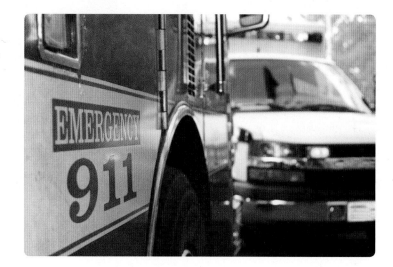

- Another trained responder or EMS personnel take over.

- You are too exhausted to continue.

- The scene becomes unsafe.

# Obtaining Consent to Help

Before giving first aid care, you must obtain **consent** (permission) from the injured or ill person (or the person's parent or guardian if the person is a minor) (Figure 1-2). To obtain consent:

- State your name.

- State the type and level of training that you have (such as training in first aid or CPR).

- Explain what you think is wrong.

- Explain what you plan to do.

- Ask if you may help.

With this information, an ill or injured person can grant his or her consent for care. Someone who is unresponsive, confused or mentally impaired may not be able to grant consent. In these cases, the law assumes the person would give consent if he or she were able to do so. This is called **implied consent**. Implied consent also applies when a minor needs emergency medical assistance and the minor's parent or guardian is not present.

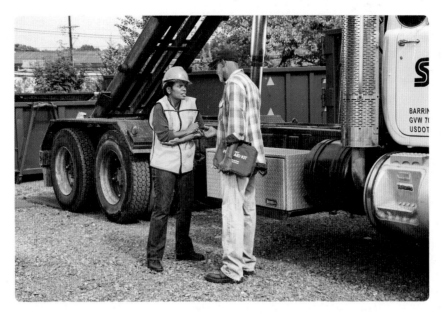

**Figure 1-2.** Obtain consent before giving care.

An injured or ill person may refuse care, even if he or she desperately needs it. A parent or guardian also may refuse care for a minor in his or her care. You must honor the person's wishes. Explain to the person why you believe care is necessary, but do not touch or give care to the person if care was refused. If you believe the person's condition is life threatening, call EMS personnel to evaluate the situation. If the person gives consent initially but then withdraws it, stop giving care and call for EMS personnel if you have not already done so.

If you do not speak the same language as the injured or ill person, obtaining consent may be challenging. Find out if someone else at the scene can serve as a translator. If a translator is not available, do your best to communicate with the person by using gestures and facial expressions. When you call 9-1-1 or the designated emergency number, explain that you are having difficulty communicating with the person, and tell the dispatcher which language you believe the person speaks. The dispatcher may have someone available who can help with communication.

# Lowering the Risk for Infection

Giving first aid care is a hands-on activity. Providing this care can put you in close contact with another person's body fluids (such as saliva, mucus, vomit or blood), which may contain **pathogens** (harmful microorganisms that can cause disease). Pathogens can be spread from person to person through direct or indirect contact. In direct transmission, the pathogen is passed from one person to another through close physical contact. In indirect transmission, the pathogen is spread by way of a contaminated surface or object.

Some pathogens that you could be exposed to when providing first aid care pose particular risk because of their long-term effects on your health if you become infected (Box 1-6).

- **Bloodborne pathogens** are spread when blood from an infected person enters the bloodstream of a person who is not infected. Bloodborne illnesses that are of particular concern include human immunodeficiency virus (HIV) infection and hepatitis B, C and D. Fortunately, although bloodborne pathogens can cause serious illnesses, they are not easily transmitted and are not spread by casual contact. Remember, for infection to occur, an infected person's blood must enter your bloodstream. This could happen through direct or indirect contact with an infected person's blood if it comes in contact with your eyes, the mucous membranes that line your mouth and nose, or an area of broken skin on your body.

You could also become infected if you stick yourself with a contaminated needle (a "needlestick injury") or cut yourself with broken glass that has been contaminated with blood.

- **Airborne pathogens** are pathogens that are expelled into the air when an infected person breathes, coughs or sneezes. Infection spreads when a person who is not infected inhales respiratory droplets containing the pathogens. Examples of airborne illnesses include tuberculosis and influenza.

---

## Box 1-6. **Bloodborne and Airborne Illnesses**

Although the risk of catching a disease when giving first aid care is very low, whenever you give care, there is the potential to be exposed to an infectious disease. Of particular concern are diseases that are not easily treated and can have long-term effects on your health, should you become infected. Using personal protective equipment (PPE) reduces your risk for catching an infectious disease significantly.

### Bloodborne Illnesses

- **HIV** is a virus that invades and destroys the cells that help us to fight off infections. A person who is infected with HIV may look and feel healthy for many years. However, during this time, the virus is breaking down the person's immune system. Eventually, a person who is infected with HIV may develop acquired immunodeficiency syndrome (AIDS). A person with AIDS is unable to fight off infections that a healthy person would be able to resist or control. The person dies from one of these infections. Although medications have been developed to help slow the progression of HIV infection, currently there is no cure.

- **Hepatitis** is inflammation of the liver, an organ that performs many vital functions for the body. There are many different types and causes of hepatitis. Hepatitis B, hepatitis C and hepatitis D are caused by infection with bloodborne viruses. Chronic infection with the viruses that cause hepatitis B, C or D can lead to liver failure, liver cancer and other serious conditions.

### Airborne Illnesses

- **Tuberculosis** is a bacterial infection of the lungs that is spread through the air from one person to another. Although tuberculosis primarily affects the lungs, it can also affect the bones, brain, kidneys and other organs. If not treated, tuberculosis can be fatal. Treatment is complex and involves taking many different medications over an extended period of time.

---

## Limiting Your Exposure to Pathogens

There are two main steps you can take to limit your exposure to pathogens and your risk for contracting a communicable disease while giving first aid care: use personal protective equipment (PPE) and wash your hands after giving care.

# Personal Protective Equipment

**Personal protective equipment (PPE)** is equipment used to prevent pathogens from contaminating your skin, mucous membranes or clothing. Articles of PPE that are commonly used when giving first aid care include latex-free disposable gloves and CPR breathing barriers. Face masks and protective eyewear are other types of PPE that may be used in a first aid situation.

**Safety First!** Be prepared by having a first aid kit handy and adequately stocked with PPE. You can also carry a keychain kit containing a pair of latex-free disposable gloves and a breathing barrier so that you always have this equipment readily available.

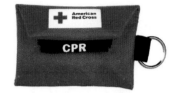

## Latex-Free Disposable Gloves

Disposable gloves are meant to be worn once and then discarded. Never clean or reuse disposable gloves. Disposable gloves should fit properly and be free of rips or tears. Wear latex-free disposable gloves:

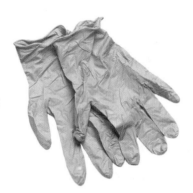

- When providing care, especially whenever there is a possibility that you will come in contact with a person's blood or other potentially infectious materials.

- When there is a break in the skin on your own hands (cover any cuts, scrapes or sores before putting on the gloves).

- When you must handle items or surfaces soiled with blood or other potentially infectious materials.

When you are wearing gloves, try to limit how much you touch other surfaces with your gloved hands. Pathogens from your soiled gloves can transfer to other items or surfaces that you touch, putting the next person who handles the item or touches the surface at risk for infection. If possible, remove soiled gloves and replace them with a clean pair before touching other surfaces or equipment in your first aid kit. When you are finished providing care, remove your gloves using proper technique to avoid contaminating your own skin (Skill Sheet 1-1), dispose of the gloves properly and wash your hands. When multiple people are in need of care, remove your gloves, wash your hands and replace your gloves with a clean pair before assisting the next person.

**Safety First!** Because many people are allergic to latex, the American Red Cross recommends the use of latex-free disposable gloves. Nitrile gloves are preferred over other types of latex-free disposable gloves, such as those made of vinyl.

## CPR Breathing Barriers

CPR **breathing barriers** are used to protect you from contact with saliva and other body fluids, such as blood, as you give rescue breaths. Breathing barriers also protect you from breathing the air that the person exhales. The most basic and portable type of breathing barrier is a **face shield**, a flat piece of thin plastic that you place over the person's face, with the opening over the person's mouth. The opening contains a filter or a valve that protects you from coming into contact with the person's body fluids and exhaled air. A **pocket mask** is a transparent, flexible device that creates a tight seal over the person's nose and mouth to allow you to give rescue breaths without making mouth-to-mouth contact or inhaling exhaled air. Breathing barriers sized specifically for children and infants are available. Always use equipment that is sized appropriately for the injured or ill person.

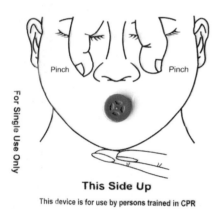

**This Side Up**

This device is for use by persons trained in CPR

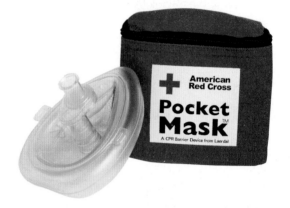

## Hand Washing

Wash your hands thoroughly with soap and warm running water when you have finished giving care, even if you wore disposable gloves. Wash for a minimum of 20 seconds and make sure to cover all surfaces of both hands: your wrists, the palms and backs of your hands, in between your fingers and underneath your fingernails.

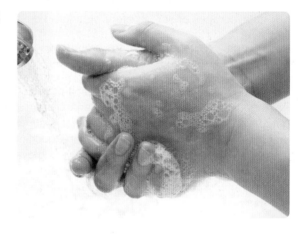

If soap and water are not available, you may use an alcohol-based hand sanitizer to decontaminate your hands. When using an alcohol-based hand sanitizer, use the amount of product recommended by the manufacturer. Rub it thoroughly over all surfaces of your hands, including your nails and in between your fingers, until the product dries. Wash your hands with soap and water as soon as you have access to hand-washing facilities.

**Safety First!** Alcohol-based hand sanitizers may not be as effective if your hands are visibly soiled with dirt or body fluids. In addition, although using an alcohol-based hand sanitizer properly will reduce the number of pathogens on your hands, it may not eliminate all pathogens. For these reasons, always wash your hands with soap and water as soon as you can, even if you used an alcohol-based hand sanitizer!

# Cleaning and Disinfecting Surfaces and Equipment

Reusable equipment and surfaces that have been contaminated by blood or other potentially infectious materials need to be properly cleaned and disinfected before the equipment is put back into service or the area is reopened. Clean and disinfect surfaces and equipment as soon as possible after the incident occurs. Remember to wear appropriate PPE.

If blood or other potentially infectious materials have spilled on the floor or another surface, prevent others from accessing the area. If the spill contains a sharp object (e.g., shards of broken glass), do not pick the object up with your hands. Instead, use tongs, a disposable scoop and scraper, or two pieces of cardboard to remove and dispose of the object. Wipe up or absorb the spill using absorbent towels or a solidifier (a fluid-absorbing powder). After wiping up the spill, flood the area with a freshly mixed disinfectant solution of approximately 1½ cups of bleach to 1 gallon of water (1 part bleach to 9 parts water, or about a 10 percent solution). When using a bleach solution, always ensure good ventilation and wear gloves and eye protection. Let the bleach solution stand on the surface for at least 10 minutes. Then use clean absorbent materials (such as paper towels) to wipe up the disinfectant solution and dry the area. Dispose of all materials used to clean up the blood spill in a labeled biohazard container. If a biohazard container is not available, place the soiled materials in a sealable plastic bag or a plastic container with a lid, seal the container and dispose of it properly.

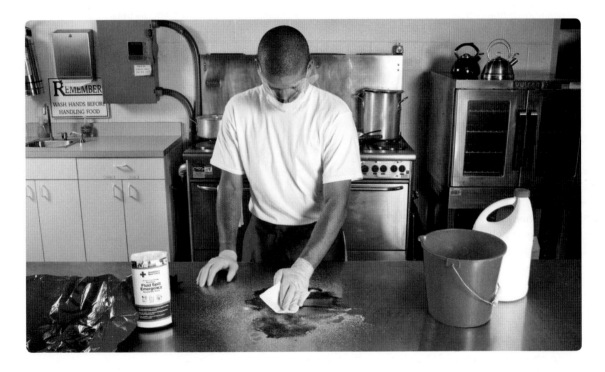

# Handling an Exposure Incident

If another person's blood or other potentially infectious material comes into contact with your eyes, the mucous membranes of your mouth or nose, or an opening or break in your skin, or if you experience a needlestick injury, then you have been involved in an exposure incident. In the event of an exposure incident, follow these steps immediately:

- Decontaminate the exposed area. If your skin was exposed, wash the contaminated area with soap and water. For splashes into your mouth or nose, flush the area with water. For splashes into the eyes, irrigate the eyes with water, saline or a sterile irrigant for 15 to 20 minutes.

- Report the exposure incident to EMS personnel or your healthcare provider.

- If the exposure incident occurred in a workplace setting, notify your supervisor and follow your company's exposure control plan for reporting the incident and receiving post-exposure follow-up care.

# Taking Action: The Emergency Action Steps

In any emergency situation, there are three simple steps to take to guide your actions. If you ever feel nervous or confused, remember these three emergency action steps to get you back on track:

1. **CHECK** the scene and the person.

2. **CALL** 9-1-1 or the designated emergency number.

3. **CARE** for the person.

## Check

First, check the scene. Then check the person.

### Check the Scene

Before rushing to help an injured or ill person, conduct a **scene size-up** and form an initial impression. Try to answer these questions:

- **Is the scene safe to enter?** Check for hazards that could jeopardize your safety or the safety of bystanders, such as fire, downed electrical wires, spilled chemicals, an unstable building or traffic. Do not enter bodies of water unless you are specifically trained to perform in-water rescues (Box 1-7). Avoid entering confined areas with poor ventilation and places where natural gas, propane or other substances could explode. Do not enter the scene if there is evidence of criminal activity or the person is hostile or threatening suicide. If these or other dangers threaten, stay at a safe distance and call 9-1-1 or the designated emergency number immediately. Once professional responders make the scene safe, you can offer your assistance as appropriate.

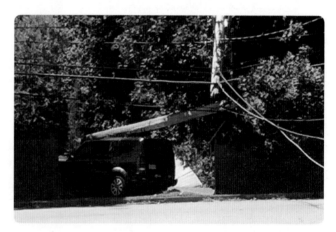

- **What happened?** Take note of anything that might tell you the cause of the emergency. If the person is unresponsive and there are no witnesses, your check of the scene may offer the only clues as to what happened. Use your senses to detect anything out of the ordinary, such as broken glass, a spilled bottle of medication or an unusual smell or sound. Keep in mind that the injured or ill person may not be exactly where he or she was when the injury or illness occurred—someone may have moved the person, or the person may have moved in an attempt to get help.

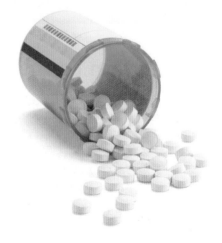

- **How many people are involved?** Look carefully for more than one injured or ill person. A person who is moving or making noise or who has very visible injuries will likely attract your attention right away, but there may be a person who is silent and not moving or a person obscured by debris or wreckage that you do not notice at first. It also is easy to overlook a small child or an infant. In an emergency with more than one injured or ill person, you may need to prioritize care (in other words, decide who needs help first).

# Box 1-7. **Reach or Throw, Don't Go!**

Never go into water or onto ice in an attempt to rescue a person who is in trouble. Instead, get help from a trained responder, such as a lifeguard, to get the person out of the water as quickly and safely as possible.

Reaching and throwing assists are the safest assists for responders who are not professionally trained lifeguards to use to help a person who is in trouble in the water. When doing a reaching or throwing assist:

- Talk to the person and let the person know help is coming.

- Tell the person what he or she can do to help with the rescue, such as grasping a line or other floating device. Use gestures to communicate with the person if it is too noisy or if the person is too far away to hear.

- Encourage the person to move toward safety by kicking his or her legs or stroking with his or her arms. Some people are able to reach safety by themselves with calm encouragement from a person on the deck or shore.

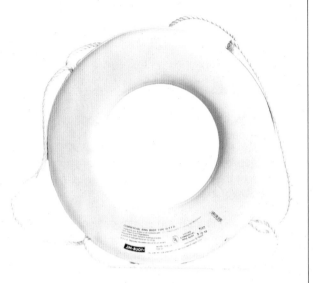

**Reaching assist.** To do a reaching assist, use any available object that will extend your reach and give the person something to grab onto (such as a pole, an oar or paddle, a branch or a towel). Extend the object to the person, tell him or her to hold on, and pull the person to safety. If no equipment is available and you are close enough, you may be able to perform a reaching assist by extending your arm to the person. You can also perform a reaching assist from a position within the water by extending an arm or a leg to the person, if you are already in the water and you have something secure to hold onto.

**Throwing assist.** A throwing assist involves throwing a floating object to the person so that he or she can grasp it and be pulled to safety. A floating object with a line attached (such as a ring buoy) is ideal for a throwing assist; however, a line or an object that floats (such as a life jacket or cooler) can also be used alone.

**Wading assist.** A wading assist involves wading into the water and using a reaching assist to help pull the person to safety. Only use a wading assist in water that is less than chest deep. If a current or soft bottom makes wading dangerous, do not enter the water. For your own safety, wear a life jacket if one is available and take something to extend to the person, such as a ring buoy, branch, pole or paddle.

---

- **What is your initial impression about the nature of the person's illness or injury?** Before you reach the person, try to form an initial impression about the person's condition and what is wrong. For example, does the person seem alert, or confused or sleepy? Look at the person's skin—does it appear to be its normal color, or does it seem pale, ashen (gray) or flushed? Is the person moving, or motionless? Does the person have any immediately identifiable injuries? Look for signs of a life-threatening illness or injury, such as loss of consciousness, trouble breathing or severe bleeding. If you see severe, life-threatening bleeding, use the resources available to you to control the bleeding as soon as possible (see Chapter 6).

- **Is anyone else available to help?** Take note of bystanders who can be of assistance. A bystander who was there when the emergency occurred or who knows the injured or ill person may be able to provide valuable information about the situation or the person. Bystanders can also assist in other ways, such as by calling 9-1-1 or the designated emergency number, waiting for EMS personnel and leading them to the site of the emergency, getting needed items (such as an AED and first aid kit), controlling crowds and reassuring the injured or ill person.

## Check the Person

When you reach the person, you can conduct a more thorough check to determine what is wrong and what care is needed.

If the person is awake and responsive, obtain consent and then begin to gather additional information about the nature of the person's illness or injury. Chapter 2 provides more detail about how to check a person who is responsive.

If the person appears to be unresponsive, shout, using the person's name if you know it. If there is no response, tap the person's shoulder (if the person is an adult or child) or the bottom of the person's foot (if the person is an infant) and shout again while checking for normal breathing. Check for responsiveness and breathing for no more than 5 to 10 seconds. If the person does not respond to you in any way (such as by moving, opening his or her eyes, or moaning) and the person is not breathing or is only gasping, the person is unresponsive. If the person responds and is breathing normally, the person is responsive, but may not be fully awake. Give care according to the conditions that you find and your level of knowledge and training (see Chapter 2).

Unresponsiveness, trouble breathing and severe bleeding are all signs of a life-threatening emergency. If your initial check of the person reveals these or any other life-threatening conditions (see Box 1-5), make sure that someone calls 9-1-1 or the designated emergency number right away. Also have someone bring an AED and a first aid kit, if these items are available.

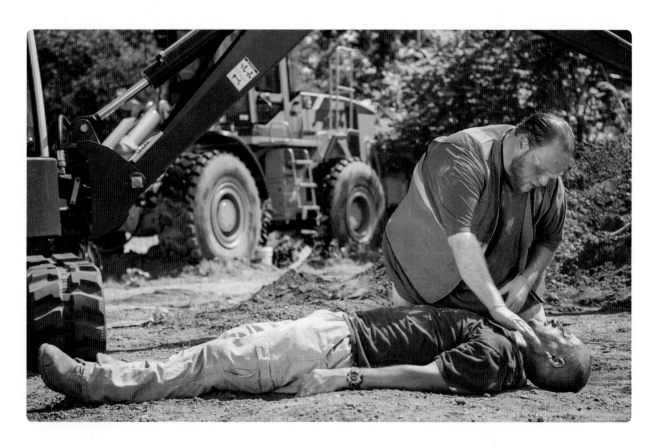

# Call

If you decide it is necessary to summon EMS personnel (see Box 1-5), make the call quickly and return to the person. If possible, ask someone else to make the call so that you can begin giving care. The person making the call should be prepared to give the dispatcher the following information:

- The location of the emergency (the address, or nearby intersections or landmarks if the address is not known)

- The nature of the emergency (e.g., whether police, fire or medical assistance is needed)

- The telephone number of the phone being used

- A description of what happened

- The number of injured or ill people

- What help, if any, has been given so far, and by whom

The caller should stay on the phone until the dispatcher tells him or her it is all right to hang up. The dispatcher may need more information. Many dispatchers also are trained to give first aid and CPR instructions over the phone, which can be helpful if you are unsure of what to do or need to be reminded of the proper care steps.

If you are alone and there is no one to send to call 9-1-1 or the designated emergency number, you may need to decide whether to call first or give care first (Box 1-8). Call First situations are likely to be cardiac arrest. In cardiac arrest, the priority is getting help on the scene as soon as possible because early access to EMS personnel and an AED increases the person's chances for survival. Care First situations include breathing emergencies and severe life-threatening bleeding. In these situations, there are immediate actions that you can take at the scene that may prevent the person's condition from worsening. After you take these actions, call 9-1-1 or the designated emergency number to get advanced medical help on the way.

## Box 1-8. Call First or Care First?

Most of the time, you will call first and then give care. But if you are alone, you may have to decide whether to call first or care first.

If you are ALONE:

**CALL First** (call 9-1-1 or the designated emergency number before giving care) for:

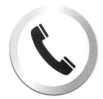

- Any person about 12 years or older who is unresponsive.

- A child or an infant whom you witnessed suddenly collapse.

- An unresponsive child or infant known to have heart problems.

**CARE First** (give immediate care, then call 9-1-1 or the designated emergency number) for:

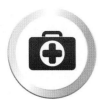

- An unresponsive infant or child younger than about 12 years whom you did not see collapse.

- A person who is choking.

- A person who is experiencing a severe allergic reaction (anaphylaxis) and has an epinephrine auto injector.

- A person who has severe, life-threatening bleeding.

# Care

The final emergency action step is to give care according to the conditions that you find and your level of knowledge and training. Follow these general guidelines:

- Do no further harm.

- Monitor the person's breathing and level of consciousness.

- Help the person rest in the most comfortable position.

- Keep the person from getting chilled or overheated.

- Reassure the person by telling the person that you will help and that EMS personnel have been called (if appropriate).

- Give care consistent with your knowledge and training as needed, and continue to watch for changes in the person's condition.

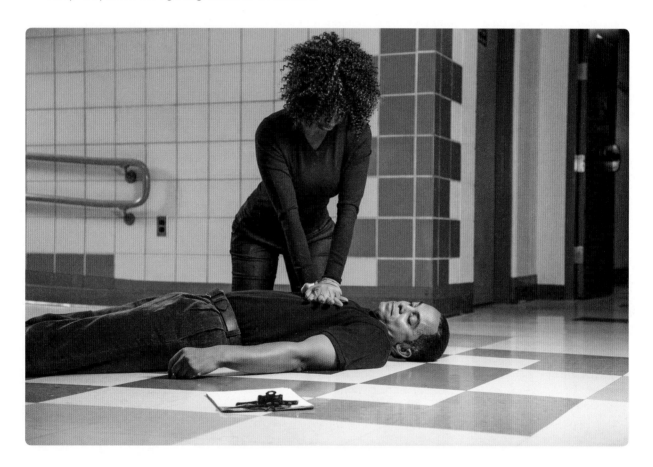

Generally speaking, you should avoid moving an injured or ill person to give care. Unnecessary movement can cause additional injury and pain and may complicate the person's recovery. However, under the following three conditions, it would be appropriate to move an injured or ill person:

- You must move the person to protect him or her from immediate danger (such as fire, flood or poisonous gas). However, you should only attempt this if you can reach the person and remove him or her from the area without endangering yourself.

- You must move the person to reach another person who may have a more serious injury or illness.

- You must move the person to give proper care. For example, it may be necessary to move a person who needs CPR onto a hard, flat surface.

If you must move the person, use one of the techniques described in Appendix A, Emergency Moves.

If the person does not have a life-threatening illness or injury, you may decide to take the injured or ill person to a medical facility yourself instead of calling for EMS personnel. Never transport a person yourself if the person has or may develop a life-threatening condition, if you are unsure of the nature of the injury or illness, or if the trip may aggravate the injury or cause additional injury.

If you decide it is safe to transport the person yourself, be sure you know the quickest route to the nearest medical facility capable of handling emergency care. Ask someone to come with you to help keep the person comfortable and monitor the person for changes in condition so that you can focus on driving. Remember to obey traffic laws. No one will benefit if you are involved in a motor-vehicle collision or get a speeding ticket on your way to the medical facility.

Discourage an injured or ill person from driving him- or herself to the hospital. An injury may restrict movement, or the person may become faint. The sudden onset of pain may be distracting. Any of these conditions can make driving dangerous for the person, passengers, other drivers and pedestrians.

# Removing Latex-Free Disposable Gloves

1.  Pinch the palm side of one glove on the outside near your wrist.

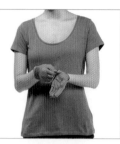

2.  Pull the glove toward your fingertips, turning it inside out as you pull it off your hand.

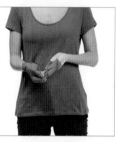

3.  Hold the glove in the palm of your other (still-gloved) hand.

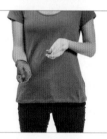

4.  Carefully slip two fingers under the wrist of the other glove. Avoid touching the outside of the glove.

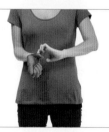

5.  Pull the glove toward your fingertips, turning it inside out as you pull it off your hand. The other glove is now contained inside.

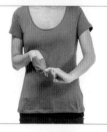

6.  Dispose of the gloves properly and wash your hands.

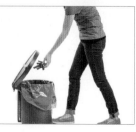

# 2

# CHECKING AN INJURED OR ILL PERSON

**B**efore you can give first aid care, you need to gather information that will guide your next actions. Your first goal is to identify and care for any life-threatening conditions. If the person does not appear to have any life-threatening conditions, you can check the person for other types of injuries or conditions that may require care. The observations you make and the information you gather will help you to better understand the nature of the emergency and give appropriate, effective care.

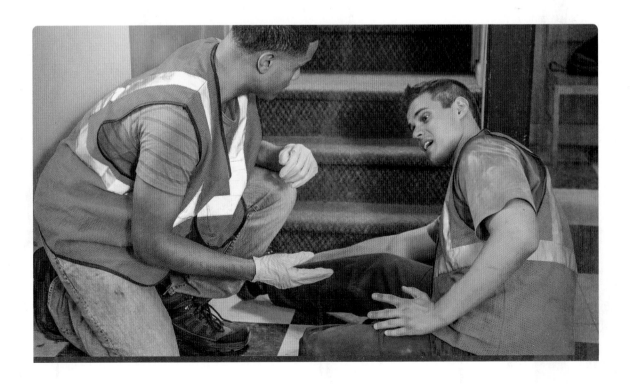

# Checking a Responsive Person

After sizing up the scene, if your initial check of the person reveals that he or she is responsive and awake, start by introducing yourself and getting consent to give care. If the person does not have any immediately obvious life-threatening conditions, begin to gather additional information about the nature of the person's illness or injury by interviewing the person and checking him or her from head to toe (Skill Sheet 2-1). Tailor your approach to the age of the person, as well as to any special circumstances (Box 2-1).

---

## Box 2-1. Strategies for Gathering Information Effectively

Being able to communicate and interact effectively with the person who is injured or ill can increase the person's comfort level with you, and makes it more likely that you will be able to get the information you need in order to provide appropriate care.

### When the Injured or Ill Person Is a Child

- If the child's parent or guardian is present, remember to get the parent's or guardian's consent to give care.

- Be aware that children often take emotional cues from the adults around them. If the child sees that adults are upset, the child's anxiety and panic may increase. Stay calm, and encourage the child's parent or guardian to do the same.

- The child's parent or guardian can be a valuable source of information if the child is not able to speak for him- or herself. However, if the child is old enough to understand and answer your questions, speak directly to the child using age-appropriate language, rather than addressing your questions to the parent or guardian.

- If the care you need to provide will cause discomfort or pain, describe what the child can expect to feel in terms the child can understand. Never make promises or statements that you cannot support (e.g., do not say that something will not hurt if it will).

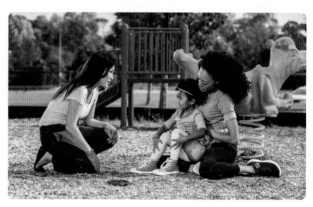

- Take into consideration the child's developmental stage.

  o **Infants (birth to 1 year).** Infants older than 6 months often show "stranger anxiety." They may turn away from you, cry and cling to their parent. If possible, check the infant while he or she is held or seated in the parent's lap.

  o **Toddlers (1 to 3 years).** A toddler may also become anxious if separated from his or her parent. If possible, give the toddler a few minutes to get used to you before attempting to check him or her, and check the toddler while he or she is seated in the parent's lap. Allowing the toddler to hold a special toy or blanket can be comforting.

*(Continued)*

○ **Preschoolers (3 to 5 years).** Preschoolers are naturally curious. Allowing the child to examine items, such as bandages, can distract the child while you are checking him or her and providing care. If time permits, showing the child what you are going to do on a stuffed animal or doll can help the child understand how you will care for him or her. Preschoolers often have a fear of body mutilation and may become very upset if they can see the results of an injury (e.g., a bleeding wound or a deformed broken limb).

○ **School-age children (5 to 12 years).** Children of this age are usually comfortable speaking with adults. They are able to understand what is happening and follow directions. Answer the child's questions honestly, and let the child know if you are going to do anything that might cause pain.

○ **Adolescents (12 to 20 years).** Adolescents may feel embarrassed and self-conscious about their changing bodies. Respect their modesty, and be aware that an adolescent may be more comfortable being checked by a person of the same gender.

# When the Injured or Ill Person Is an Older Adult

- Pay attention to how the person introduces him- or herself. If the person gives a last name, consider addressing the person more formally (e.g., "Mr. Johnson" rather than "Bill") as a sign of respect.

- A family member, caregiver or other person who knows the older adult well can be a valuable source of information if the older adult is not able to speak for him- or herself. However, if the older adult is able to understand and answer your questions, speak directly to him or her, rather than addressing your questions to others who might be present.

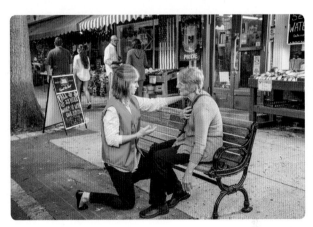

- Speak clearly and loudly enough for the person to hear you, but do not shout. If the person does not seem to understand what you are saying, change your words, not the volume of your voice, unless you spoke too softly.

- When interviewing the person, avoid rushing. Allow the person enough time to process your questions and respond.

- Be aware that in older people, the signs and symptoms of a medical emergency may be very general and nonspecific, and they may not even be noticeable to someone who does not know the person well. General signs and symptoms that could indicate a medical emergency in an older adult include headache, a change in the person's usual level of activity, a change in mental status (such as agitation, the new onset of confusion, or increased confusion in a person who is already confused), lethargy (extreme drowsiness or sleepiness) and difficulty sleeping.

- Many older adults have impaired hearing, vision or both. If the person seems confused, make sure the "confusion" is not just the result of being unable to hear you or see you clearly. If the person normally wears a hearing aid, make sure it is in place and turned on. If the person usually wears glasses, make sure he or she has them on.

*(Continued)*

## Box 2-1. continued

# When the Injured or Ill Person Has a Disability

- A family member, caregiver or other person who knows the injured or ill person well can be a valuable source of information if the person is not able to speak for him- or herself. However, if the person is able to understand and answer your questions, speak directly to him or her, rather than addressing your questions to others who might be present.

- A person with a disability may use a service animal. Be aware that service animals are trained to protect their owners, and both the service animal and the person may become anxious if they are separated. Allow the service animal to stay with the person if possible.

- If the person wears an assistive device (e.g., a leg brace), do not remove the device when you are examining the person.

- If the person has an intellectual disability:
  - Address the person as you would any other person in his or her age group. If the person does not seem to understand you, rephrase your statement or question in simpler terms.
  - Be aware that being injured or becoming suddenly ill may make the person very upset, anxious or fearful. Take time to explain who you are and what you intend to do, and reassure the person.

- If the person has impaired hearing:
  - Approach the person from the front.
  - Hearing-impaired people who know how to read lips rely on watching your mouth move. Position yourself so that the person can see your mouth and facial expressions. Pronounce your words slowly and clearly, and speak in short sentences.
  - If the person does not seem to understand what you are saying, change your words, not the volume of your voice, unless you spoke too softly. Shouting sometimes causes the person more distress and he or she still may not understand what you are trying to say.
  - Use gestures or written messages as necessary to make your meaning clear.

- If the person has impaired vision:
  - Speak in a normal voice. It is not necessary to shout.
  - As you provide care, describe what you are doing.

# When the Injured or Ill Person Speaks a Different Language

- Speak in a normal voice. It is not necessary to shout.

- Find out if any bystanders speak the person's language and can assist by translating.

- Do your best to communicate nonverbally, using gestures and facial expressions.

- When you call 9-1-1 or the designated emergency number, explain that you are having difficulty communicating with the person, and tell the dispatcher which language you believe the person speaks. The dispatcher may have someone available who can help with communication.

**Safety First!** Sometimes people who have been injured or become suddenly ill may act strangely; be uncooperative; or become violent, angry or aggressive. This behavior can be the result of the injury or illness or other factors, such as the effects of drugs, alcohol or medications. Do not take this behavior personally. If you feel threatened by the person's behavior, move away from the person to safety and call 9-1-1 or the designated emergency number, if you have not already done so.

# Interviewing the Person

Begin by asking the person's name, and use it when you speak to the person. Position yourself at eye level with the person and speak clearly, calmly and in a friendly manner, using age-appropriate language. Try to provide as much privacy as possible for the person while you are conducting the interview, and keep the interview brief. The mnemonic SAMPLE (Figure 2-1) can help you remember what you should ask about. If possible, write down the information you learn during the interview or, preferably, have someone else write it down for you. Be sure to give the information to emergency medical services (EMS) personnel when they arrive. It may help them to determine the type of medical care that the person should receive.

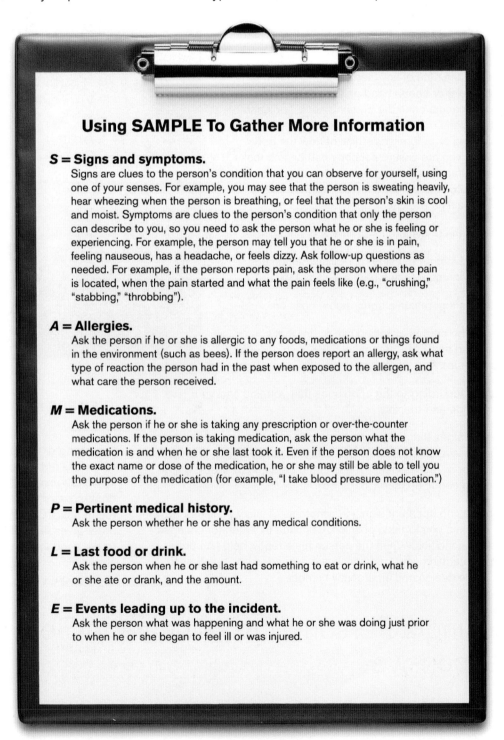

### Using SAMPLE To Gather More Information

**S = Signs and symptoms.**
Signs are clues to the person's condition that you can observe for yourself, using one of your senses. For example, you may see that the person is sweating heavily, hear wheezing when the person is breathing, or feel that the person's skin is cool and moist. Symptoms are clues to the person's condition that only the person can describe to you, so you need to ask the person what he or she is feeling or experiencing. For example, the person may tell you that he or she is in pain, feeling nauseous, has a headache, or feels dizzy. Ask follow-up questions as needed. For example, if the person reports pain, ask the person where the pain is located, when the pain started and what the pain feels like (e.g., "crushing," "stabbing," "throbbing").

**A = Allergies.**
Ask the person if he or she is allergic to any foods, medications or things found in the environment (such as bees). If the person does report an allergy, ask what type of reaction the person had in the past when exposed to the allergen, and what care the person received.

**M = Medications.**
Ask the person if he or she is taking any prescription or over-the-counter medications. If the person is taking medication, ask the person what the medication is and when he or she last took it. Even if the person does not know the exact name or dose of the medication, he or she may still be able to tell you the purpose of the medication (for example, "I take blood pressure medication.")

**P = Pertinent medical history.**
Ask the person whether he or she has any medical conditions.

**L = Last food or drink.**
Ask the person when he or she last had something to eat or drink, what he or she ate or drank, and the amount.

**E = Events leading up to the incident.**
Ask the person what was happening and what he or she was doing just prior to when he or she began to feel ill or was injured.

**Figure 2-1.** The mnemonic SAMPLE can help you remember what to ask the injured or ill person.

Other people at the scene may be able to provide useful information as well. They may have witnessed what happened. If there are people at the scene who know the injured or ill person well (such as family members or friends), they may also be able to provide information about the person's medical history, if he or she is not able to do so (for example, because of the effects of the injury or illness).

## Checking from Head to Toe

Next, check the person from head to toe. Before beginning the check, tell the person what you are going to do. Then check the person in a methodical way. Check one part of the body at a time, moving straight down the body from head to toe, and then checking the arms.

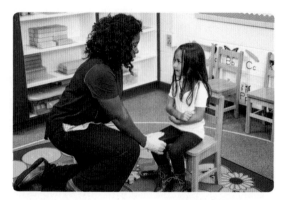

As you check, take note of any medical identification tags, such as a bracelet or sports band on the person's wrist or ankle, or a necklace around the person's neck. Look and gently feel for signs of injury, such as bleeding, cuts, burns, bruising, swelling or deformities. Think of how the body usually looks. If you are unsure if a body part or limb looks injured, check it against the opposite limb or the other side of the body. Watch the person's face for expressions of discomfort or pain as you check for injuries.

If you detect signs or symptoms of illness or injury:

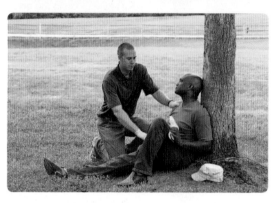

- Determine whether to call 9-1-1 or the designated emergency number (see Chapter 1, Box 1-5).

- Help the person rest in a comfortable position.

- Reassure the person by telling him or her that you will help and that EMS personnel have been called (if appropriate).

- Give care according to the conditions that you find and your level of knowledge and training.

- Be alert to signs that the person's condition is worsening, such as changes in level of consciousness, changes in breathing, changes in skin color or restlessness. These could be signs of shock, a life-threatening condition (see Chapter 5).

If the person has no apparent signs or symptoms of injury or illness, have him or her rest in a comfortable position. Continue to watch for changes in the person's condition. When the person feels ready, help him or her to stand up. Determine what additional care is needed and whether to call 9-1-1 or the designated emergency number.

### THE PROS KNOW.

In a young or frightened child who does not appear to have a life-threatening illness or injury, do the reverse—check from toe to head. Checking in this order gives the child a chance to get used to the process and allows him or her to see what is going on.

# Checking a Person Who Appears to Be Unresponsive

If you think an injured or ill person is unresponsive, shout to get the person's attention, using the person's name if you know it. If there is no response, tap the person's shoulder (if the person is an adult or child) or the bottom of the person's foot (if the person is an infant), and shout again while checking for normal breathing. (Isolated or infrequent gasping is not normal breathing.) Check for responsiveness and breathing for no more than 5 to 10 seconds.

# If the Person Is Responsive

If the person responds (such as by moving, opening his or her eyes or moaning) and is breathing normally, the person is responsive, but may not be fully awake. If the person is not fully awake but appears to be breathing normally, send someone to call 9-1-1 or the designated emergency number and to obtain an automated external defibrillator (AED) and first aid kit. Gather more information by interviewing bystanders (using SAMPLE as a guide; see Figure 2-1) and doing a head-to-toe check. Then roll the person onto his or her side into the recovery position (Box 2-2).

# If the Person Is Unresponsive

If the person does not respond in any way and is not breathing or is only gasping, assume cardiac arrest. Send someone to call 9-1-1 or the designated emergency number and to get an AED and first aid kit. Make sure the person is lying face-up on a firm, flat surface, such as the ground or floor. Immediately begin CPR (starting with compressions) and use an AED as soon as possible if you are trained in these skills.

Skill Sheet 2-2 summarizes how to check an injured or ill person who appears to be unresponsive.

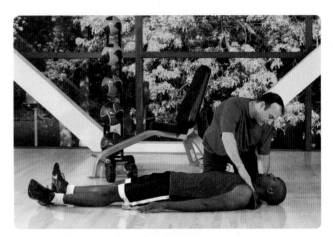

## Box 2-2. Recovery Positions

When a person is responsive but not fully awake, put the person in a recovery position if the person has no obvious signs of injury. The recovery position helps to lower the person's risk for choking and aspiration (the inhalation of foreign matter, such as saliva or vomit, into the lungs). You should also use the recovery position if a person with an injury begins to vomit, or if it is necessary to leave the person alone to call 9-1-1 or the designated emergency number.

To place an adult or child in a recovery position:

- Extend the person's arm that is closest to you above the person's head.

- Roll the person toward yourself onto his or her side, so that the person's head rests on his or her extended arm.

- Bend both of the person's knees to stabilize the body.

For an infant:

- You can place an infant on his or her side as you would an older child, or you can hold the infant in a recovery position by positioning the infant face-down along your forearm, supporting the infant's head and neck while keeping the mouth and nose clear.

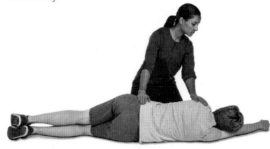

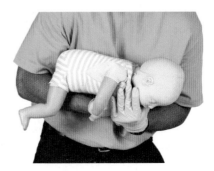

# Checking a Responsive Person

1. Interview the person (or bystanders, if necessary) using SAMPLE to get a better understanding of the situation and the nature of the person's illness or injury.

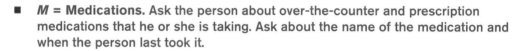

- **S = Signs and symptoms.** Take note of signs (which you can observe for yourself, using your senses) and ask the person about symptoms (feelings that only the person can describe to you, such as pain, shortness of breath or nausea).

- **A = Allergies.** Ask the person about allergies, noting causes of allergic reactions in the past and whether the allergic reaction was severe or life threatening.

- **M = Medications.** Ask the person about over-the-counter and prescription medications that he or she is taking. Ask about the name of the medication and when the person last took it.

- **P = Pertinent medical history.** Ask the person whether he or she has any medical conditions.

- **L = Last food or drink.** Ask the person when he or she last had something to eat or drink, what the person ate or drank, and how much.

- **E = Events leading up to the incident.** Ask the person what was happening and what he or she was doing just prior to when he or she began to feel ill or was injured.

2. Check each part of the body in a systematic manner from head to toe. As you check each part of the body, look and feel for signs of injury, including bleeding, cuts, burns, bruising, swelling or deformities. Note if the person has pain or discomfort or is unable or unwilling to move the body part. Also notice how the person's skin looks and feels. Is the skin pale, ashen or flushed? Does it feel moist or dry, cool or hot?

*Note: Do not ask the person to move if you suspect a head, neck or spinal injury. Do not ask the person to move any area of the body that causes discomfort or pain.*

*Note: As you check the person, take note of any medical identification tags (typically worn around the neck, wrist or ankle).*

- **Head and neck.** Check the scalp, face, ears, eyes, nose, mouth and neck for signs of injury.

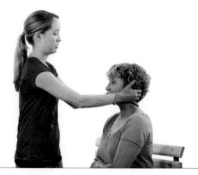

*(Continued)*

- **Shoulders.** Check the shoulders for signs of injury.

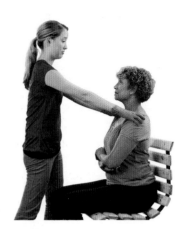

- **Chest and abdomen.** Check the chest and abdomen for signs of injury. Ask the person to take a deep breath and blow the air out. Look for trouble breathing or changes in breathing. Ask the person if he or she is experiencing pain during breathing.

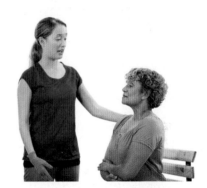

- **Hips.** Check the hips for signs of injury. Ask the person if he or she is experiencing hip pain.

- **Legs and feet.** Check each leg and foot, one at a time, for signs of injury. Ask the person to wiggle his or her toes and feet.

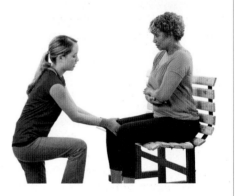

- **Arms and hands.** Check each arm and hand, one at a time, for signs of injury. Ask the person to wiggle his or her fingers and hands.

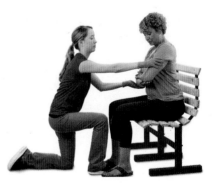

*(Continued)*

3. Provide care for any conditions found.

   ■ If your check reveals signs or symptoms of an injury or illness, call 9-1-1 or the designated emergency number (if necessary) and provide care according to the conditions that you find and your level of knowledge and training. Be alert to signs that the person's condition is worsening.

   ■ If the person has no apparent signs or symptoms of injury or illness, have him or her rest in a comfortable position. Continue to watch for changes in the person's condition.

**Skill Sheet 2-2**

# Checking a Person Who Appears to Be Unresponsive

1. **Check for responsiveness and breathing.** Shout to get the person's attention, using the person's name if you know it. If there is no response, tap the person's shoulder (if the person is an adult or child) or the bottom of the person's foot (if the person is an infant), and shout again while checking for normal breathing.

   ■ Check for responsiveness and breathing for no more than 5 to 10 seconds.

   ■ Isolated or infrequent gasping is not normal breathing.

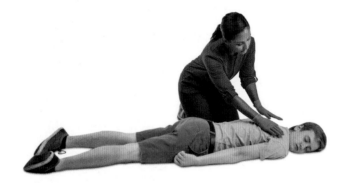 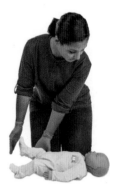

2. **If the person responds and is breathing normally but is not fully awake:**

- Send someone to call 9-1-1 or the designated emergency number and to obtain an AED and first aid kit.

- Interview bystanders (using SAMPLE as a guide) and do a head-to-toe check to gather more information.

- Place the person into the recovery position by rolling the person onto his or her side.

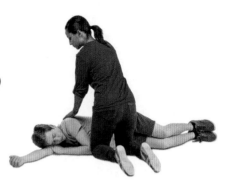

3. **If the person does not respond and is not breathing or is only gasping:**

- Send someone to call 9-1-1 or the designated emergency number and to obtain an AED and first aid kit (or, if you are alone, complete these actions yourself).

- If the person is face-down, carefully roll the person onto his or her back. If necessary, move the person to a firm, flat surface.

- Immediately begin CPR (starting with compressions) and use an AED as soon as possible, if you are trained in these skills.

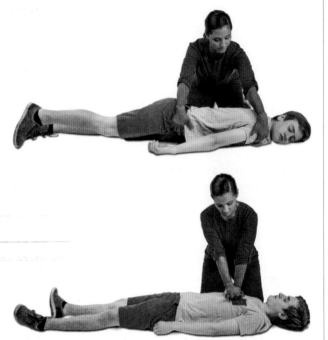

# PART 2

# First Aid for Cardiac Emergencies and Choking

# 3 CARDIAC EMERGENCIES

**L**ife-threatening cardiac emergencies often strike close to home, where we live, work and play. When you know how to recognize and respond to a cardiac emergency, the life you could save is likely to be that of someone you know—a family member, co-worker or neighbor. Because every minute counts when a person is experiencing a cardiac emergency, the person's survival often depends on lay responders acting quickly and giving appropriate care until EMS personnel arrive and take over.

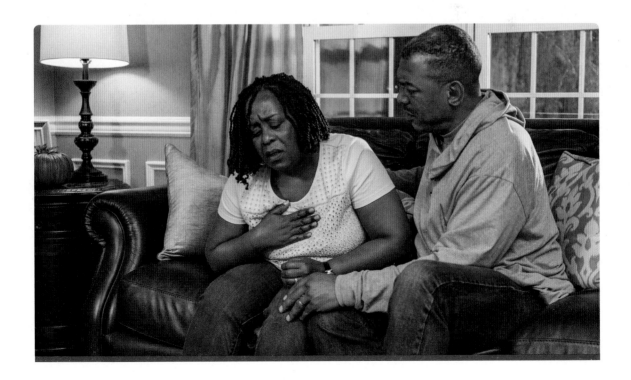

# Heart Attack

A **heart attack** occurs when blood flow to part of the heart muscle is blocked (e.g., as a result of coronary artery disease). Because the cells in the affected area of the heart muscle are not receiving the oxygen and nutrients they need, they die, causing permanent damage to the heart muscle (Figure 3-1). Seeking advanced medical care as soon as you recognize the signs and symptoms of a heart attack can minimize the damage to the heart and may save the person's life.

When a person is having a heart attack, every minute counts.

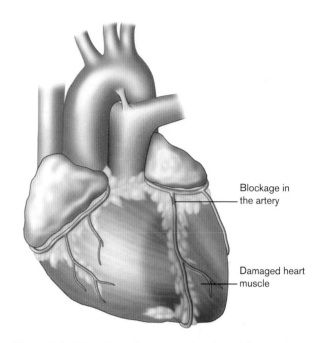

Blockage in
the artery

Damaged heart
muscle

**Figure 3-1.** A heart attack occurs when blood flow to the heart is blocked.

## Signs and Symptoms of a Heart Attack

Signs and symptoms of a heart attack vary from person to person, and can be different in women than they are in men. Even people who have had a heart attack before may not experience the same signs and symptoms if they have a second heart attack. A person who is having a heart attack may show any of the following signs and symptoms:

- Chest pain, which can range from mild to unbearable. The person may complain of pressure, squeezing, tightness, aching or heaviness in the chest. The pain or discomfort is persistent, lasting longer than 3 to 5 minutes, or going away and then coming back. It is not relieved by resting, changing position or taking medication. It may be difficult to distinguish the pain of a heart attack from the pain of indigestion, heartburn or a muscle spasm.

- Discomfort or pain that spreads to one or both arms, the back, the shoulder, the neck, the jaw or the upper part of the stomach

- Dizziness or light-headedness

- Trouble breathing, including noisy breathing, shortness of breath or breathing that is faster than normal

- Nausea or vomiting

- Pale, ashen (gray) or slightly bluish skin, especially around the face and fingers

- Sweating

- A feeling of anxiety or impending doom

- Extreme fatigue (tiredness)

- Unresponsiveness

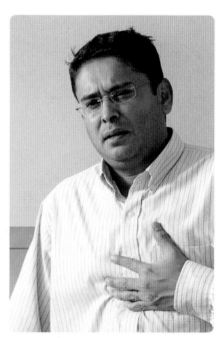

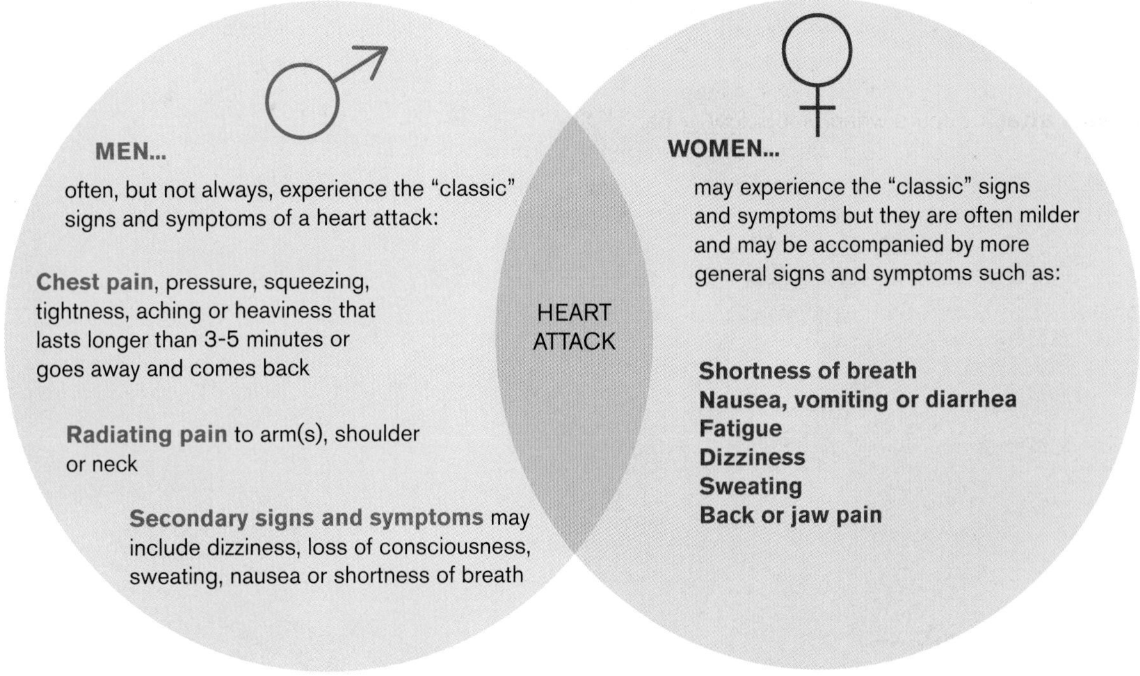

**MEN...**

often, but not always, experience the "classic" signs and symptoms of a heart attack:

**Chest pain,** pressure, squeezing, tightness, aching or heaviness that lasts longer than 3-5 minutes or goes away and comes back

**Radiating pain** to arm(s), shoulder or neck

**Secondary signs and symptoms** may include dizziness, loss of consciousness, sweating, nausea or shortness of breath

**HEART ATTACK**

**WOMEN...**

may experience the "classic" signs and symptoms but they are often milder and may be accompanied by more general signs and symptoms such as:

**Shortness of breath**
**Nausea, vomiting or diarrhea**
**Fatigue**
**Dizziness**
**Sweating**
**Back or jaw pain**

**Figure 3-2.** Men and women often experience heart attacks differently.

Although men often have the "classic" signs and symptoms of a heart attack, such as chest pain that radiates down one arm, women often have more subtle signs and symptoms or experience the signs and symptoms of a heart attack differently than men do (Figure 3-2). For example, in women, the "classic" signs and symptoms may be milder or accompanied by more general signs and symptoms such as shortness of breath; nausea or vomiting; extreme fatigue; and dizziness or light-headedness. Because these signs and symptoms are so general and nonspecific, women may experience them for hours, days or even weeks leading up to the heart attack but dismiss them as nothing out of the ordinary.

The signs and symptoms of a heart attack may also be more subtle in people with certain medical conditions, such as diabetes.

# First Aid Care for a Heart Attack

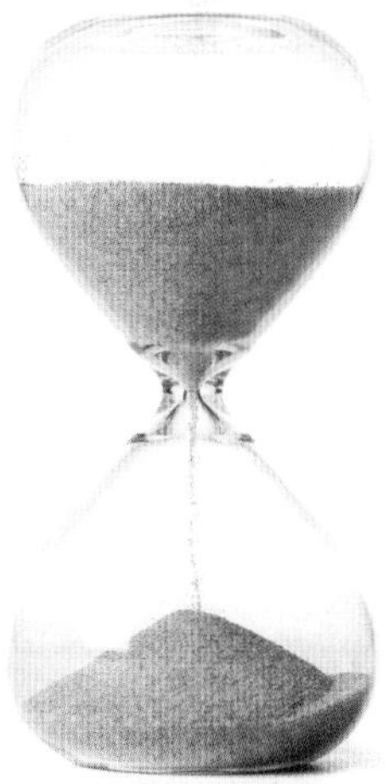

If you think that a person is having a heart attack, call 9-1-1 or the designated emergency number immediately. Trust your instincts. Many people who are having a heart attack delay seeking care because they hope they are experiencing signs and symptoms of a more minor condition that will go away with time, such as indigestion, heartburn, a muscle strain or the flu. People often worry about calling an ambulance and going to the emergency room for a "false alarm." However, most people who die of a heart attack die within 2 hours of first experiencing signs or symptoms. Even when a heart attack is not fatal, early advanced medical care can help to minimize the damage to the heart. Always seek advanced medical care as soon as signs and symptoms of a heart attack are noted.

If you think that someone might be having a heart attack, you should:

- Call 9-1-1 or the designated emergency number immediately. Never try to drive a person who is experiencing signs and symptoms of a heart attack to the hospital yourself. EMS personnel can transport the person to the hospital safely while initiating care.

- Have the person stop what he or she is doing and rest in a comfortable position to reduce the heart's need for oxygen. Many people experiencing a heart attack find it easier to breathe while sitting.

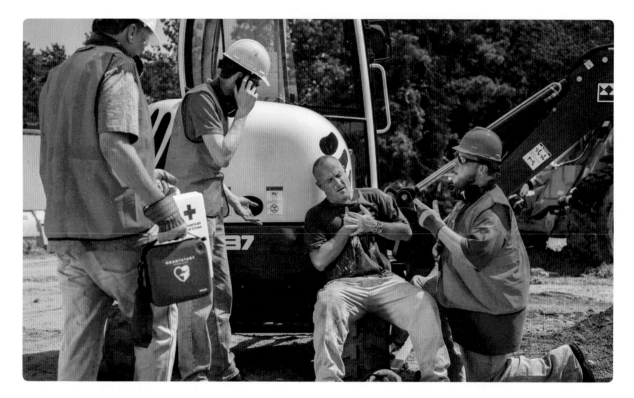

- Loosen any tight or uncomfortable clothing.

- Reassure the person. Anxiety increases the person's discomfort.

- If the person has a history of heart disease and takes a prescribed medication to relieve chest pain (e.g., nitroglycerin), offer to locate the medication and help the person to take it.

- If the person is responsive, able to chew and swallow, and allowed to have aspirin, you may offer two low-dose (81-mg) aspirin tablets or one 5-grain (325-mg) regular-strength aspirin tablet (Box 3-1).

- Closely monitor the person's condition until EMS personnel arrive and take over. Notice any changes in the person's appearance or behavior.

- If you are trained in giving CPR and using an automated external defibrillator (AED), be prepared to give CPR and use an AED if the person becomes unresponsive.

# Cardiac Arrest

Cardiac arrest is not the same as a heart attack. Remember, a heart attack occurs when blood flow to part of the heart muscle is blocked, causing part of the heart muscle to die. **Cardiac arrest**, on the other hand, occurs when the heart stops beating or beats too ineffectively to circulate blood to the brain and other vital organs. A network of special cells in the heart muscle conducts electrical impulses that coordinate contraction, causing the heart to beat rhythmically. In cardiac arrest, the electrical impulses become abnormal and chaotic. This causes the heart to lose the ability to beat rhythmically, or to stop beating altogether (Figure 3-3).

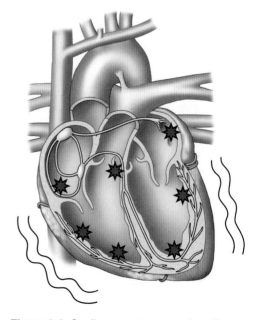

**Figure 3-3.** Cardiac arrest occurs when the electrical impulses that control the heartbeat become irregular and chaotic.

# Box 3-1. **Aspirin for a Heart Attack**

You may be able to help a person who is showing early signs and symptoms of a heart attack by offering the person an appropriate dose of aspirin. Aspirin can help to prevent blood clotting and is most effective when given soon after the onset of signs and symptoms of a heart attack. However, you should never delay calling 9-1-1 or the designated emergency number to find or offer aspirin.

Before offering aspirin, make sure the person is responsive, able to chew and swallow, and allowed to have aspirin. Ask the person:

■ Are you allergic to aspirin?

■ Do you have a stomach ulcer or stomach disease?

■ Are you taking any blood thinners, such as warfarin (Coumadin™)?

■ Have you ever been told by a healthcare provider to avoid taking aspirin?

If the person answers "no" to each of these questions, you may offer the person two low-dose (81-mg) aspirin tablets or one 5-grain (325-mg) regular-strength aspirin tablet. Have the person chew the aspirin completely. Chewing the aspirin speeds its absorption into the bloodstream.

Do not offer the person an aspirin-containing combination product meant to relieve multiple conditions, or another type of pain medication, such as acetaminophen (Tylenol®), ibuprofen (Motrin®, Advil®) or naproxen (Aleve®). These medications do not work the same way aspirin does and are not beneficial for a person who is experiencing a heart attack.

Cardiovascular disease and certain congenital heart conditions (conditions that a person is born with) can increase a person's risk for cardiac arrest. Breathing emergencies, such as choking or drowning, can also lead to cardiac arrest because if the body's supply of oxygen is interrupted, the heart soon stops beating. Every organ in the body needs a steady supply of oxygen in order to work properly, and the heart is no exception. Severe trauma, electric shock and drug overdose are other potential causes of cardiac arrest. Although cardiac arrest is more common in adults, it does occur in young people as well. The most common causes of cardiac arrest in children and infants are breathing emergencies, congenital heart disorders and trauma.

When the heart stops beating properly, the body cannot survive for long. Breathing will soon stop, and the body's organs will no longer receive the oxygen they need to function. Without oxygen, brain damage can begin in about 4 to 6 minutes, and the damage can become irreversible after about 8 to 10 minutes (Figure 3-4). Death occurs within a matter of minutes if the person does not receive immediate care.

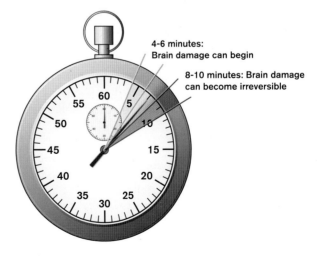

4-6 minutes:
Brain damage can begin

8-10 minutes: Brain damage can become irreversible

**Figure 3-4.** Every minute counts in cardiac arrest.

# Signs and Symptoms of Cardiac Arrest

When a person experiences cardiac arrest, you may see the person suddenly collapse. When you check the person, you will find that the person is not responsive and not breathing, or only gasping. (In an unresponsive person, isolated or infrequent gasping in the absence of normal breathing may be **agonal breaths**, which can occur even after the heart has stopped beating. Agonal breaths are not breathing and are a sign of cardiac arrest.) The person has no heartbeat.

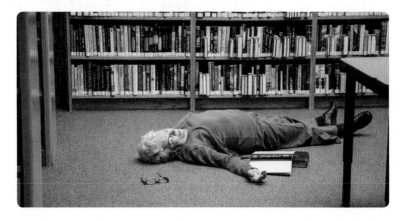

Cardiac arrest can happen suddenly and without any warning signs. When this occurs, the person is said to have experienced **sudden cardiac arrest**. People who have a history of cardiovascular disease or a congenital heart disorder are at higher risk for sudden cardiac arrest. However, sudden cardiac arrest can happen in people who appear healthy and have no known heart disease or other risk factors for the condition. A person who experiences sudden cardiac arrest is at very high risk for dying and needs immediate care.

# First Aid Care for Cardiac Arrest

When a person experiences cardiac arrest, quick action on the part of those who witness the arrest is crucial and gives the person the greatest chance for survival. The **Cardiac Chain of Survival** describes five actions that, when performed in rapid succession, increase the person's likelihood of surviving cardiac arrest (Box 3-2). In the Cardiac Chain of Survival, each link of the chain depends on, and is connected to, the other links.

Four out of every five cardiac arrests in the United States occur outside of the hospital. That means responders like you are often responsible for initiating the Cardiac Chain of Survival. When you complete the first three links in the Cardiac Chain of Survival—recognizing cardiac arrest and activating the EMS system, immediately beginning CPR and using an AED as soon as possible—you give the person the best chance for surviving the incident.

For each minute that CPR and use of an AED are delayed, the person's chance for survival is reduced by about 10 percent.

If you think that a person is in cardiac arrest:

- Have someone call 9-1-1 or the designated emergency number immediately.

- Begin CPR immediately.

- Use an AED as soon as possible.

# Box 3-2. **The Cardiac Chain of Survival**

## Adult Cardiac Chain of Survival

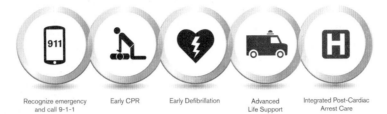

Recognize emergency and call 9-1-1 — Early CPR — Early Defibrillation — Advanced Life Support — Integrated Post-Cardiac Arrest Care

■ **Recognition of cardiac arrest and activation of the emergency medical services (EMS) system.** The sooner someone recognizes that a person is in cardiac arrest and calls 9-1-1 or the designated emergency number, the sooner people capable of providing advanced life support will arrive on the scene.

■ **Early CPR.** CPR circulates oxygen-containing blood to the brain and other vital organs, helping to prevent brain damage and death.

■ **Early defibrillation.** Defibrillation (delivery of an electrical shock using an AED) may restore an effective heart rhythm, significantly increasing the person's chances for survival.

■ **Early advanced life support.** Provided by EMS personnel at the scene and en route to the hospital, early advanced life support gives the person access to emergency medical care delivered by trained professionals.

■ **Integrated post–cardiac arrest care.** After the person is resuscitated, an interdisciplinary team of medical professionals works to stabilize the person's medical condition, minimize complications, and diagnose and treat the underlying cause of the cardiac arrest to improve survival outcomes.

## Pediatric Cardiac Chain of Survival

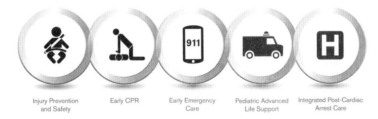

Injury Prevention and Safety — Early CPR — Early Emergency Care — Pediatric Advanced Life Support — Integrated Post-Cardiac Arrest Care

■ **Prevention.** Because cardiac arrest in children often occurs as the result of a preventable injury (such as trauma, drowning, choking or electrocution), the Pediatric Cardiac Chain of Survival has "prevention" as the first link.

■ **Early CPR.** CPR circulates oxygen-containing blood to the brain and other vital organs, helping to prevent brain damage and death.

■ **Activation of the emergency medical services (EMS) system.** The sooner someone recognizes that a person is in cardiac arrest and calls 9-1-1 or the designated emergency number, the sooner people capable of providing advanced life support will arrive on the scene.

■ **Early advanced life support.** Provided by EMS personnel at the scene and en route to the hospital, early advanced life support gives the person access to emergency medical care delivered by trained professionals.

■ **Integrated post–cardiac arrest care.** After the person is resuscitated, an interdisciplinary team of medical professionals works to stabilize the person's medical condition, minimize complications, and diagnose and treat the underlying cause of the cardiac arrest to improve survival outcomes.

# CPR

**CPR**, or cardiopulmonary resuscitation, is a skill that is used when a person is in cardiac arrest to keep oxygenated blood moving to the brain and other vital organs until advanced medical help arrives (Figure 3-5). CPR involves giving sets of 30 chest compressions followed by sets of 2 rescue breaths. When you give compressions, you press down on the person's chest. This squeezes (compresses) the heart between the breastbone (sternum) and spine, moving blood out of the heart and to the brain and other vital organs. After each compression, you must let the chest return to its normal position. This allows blood to flow back into the heart. The rescue breaths you give after each set of 30 compressions deliver a fresh supply of oxygen into the person's lungs. When you give CPR, you help to keep oxygenated blood moving throughout the body, which can buy the person some time until advanced medical help arrives.

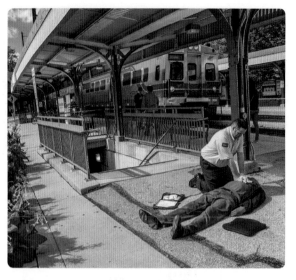

**Figure 3-5.** CPR keeps oxygen-containing blood circulating to the brain and other vital organs.

Although full CPR (compressions and rescue breaths) is preferred, if you are unable or unwilling for any reason to give full CPR, you can give **compression-only CPR** instead. In compression-only CPR, you give continuous chest compressions, with no rescue breaths. After checking the scene and the person and calling 9-1-1 or the designated emergency number, give chest compressions without stopping until another trained responder or EMS personnel take over or you notice an obvious sign of life.

## AED

While CPR can help to prevent brain damage and death by keeping oxygenated blood moving throughout the body, an AED can correct the underlying problem for some people who go into

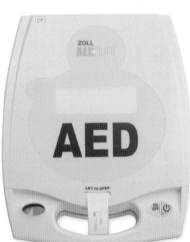

sudden cardiac arrest. Two abnormal heart rhythms in particular, **ventricular fibrillation (V-fib)** and **ventricular tachycardia (V-tach)**, can lead to sudden cardiac arrest. In V-fib, the heart muscle simply quivers (fibrillates) weakly instead of contracting strongly. In V-tach, the heart muscle contracts too fast (*tachy-* means "fast"). Both abnormal rhythms impair the heart's ability to pump and circulate blood throughout the body and are life threatening. However, in many cases, V-fib and V-tach can be corrected by an electrical shock delivered by an AED. This shock disrupts the heart's electrical activity long enough to allow the heart to spontaneously develop an effective rhythm on its own. Starting CPR immediately and using an AED as soon as possible gives the person the best chance for surviving cardiac arrest (Figure 3-6).

## THE PROS KNOW.

Many lay responders worry about hurting the person (for example, by breaking the person's ribs or breastbone) while giving CPR, but a person who is in need of CPR is clinically dead (i.e., the person has no heartbeat and is not breathing). It is very unlikely that you will injure the person while giving CPR, but even if you do, consider this: any injury you may cause is secondary when compared with the person's current circumstances, and the injury will heal with medical care and time. Remember: The worst thing to do is nothing!

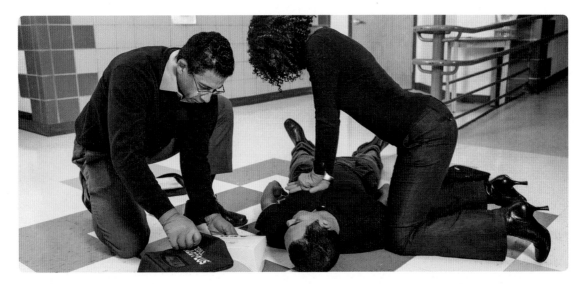

**Figure 3-6.** Immediately beginning CPR and using an AED as soon as possible gives the person the best chance for survival.

# Giving CPR

If you check a person and find that he or she is unresponsive and not breathing or only gasping, begin CPR immediately, starting with chest compressions. Proper technique is important. Skill Sheets 3-1, 3-2 and 3-3 describe step by step how to give CPR to an adult, child and infant, respectively. Table 3-1 summarizes the key differences in giving CPR to an adult, child or infant.

## Giving CPR to an Adult

First, make sure the person is lying face-up on a firm, flat surface. For example, if the person is on a soft surface like a sofa or bed, quickly move him or her to the floor before you begin. Kneel beside the person.

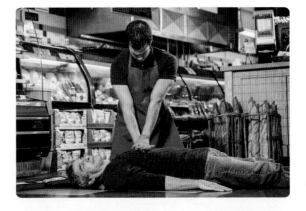

- **Position your hands.** Place the heel of one hand in the center of the person's chest on the person's breastbone (sternum). If you feel the notch at the end of the breastbone, move your hand slightly toward the person's head. Place your other hand on top of your first hand and interlace your fingers or hold them up so that your fingers are not on the person's chest. If you have arthritis in your hands, you can grasp the wrist of the hand positioned on the chest with your other hand instead. The person's clothing should not interfere with finding the proper hand position or your ability to give effective compressions. If it does, loosen or remove enough clothing to allow deep compressions in the center of the person's chest.

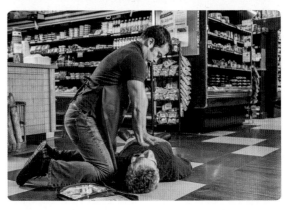

- **Give a set of 30 compressions.** Position your body so that your shoulders are directly over your hands. This will let you push on the chest using a straight up-and-down motion, which moves the most blood with each push and is also less tiring. Keeping

# TABLE 3-1 Comparison of CPR Technique in Adults, Children and Infants

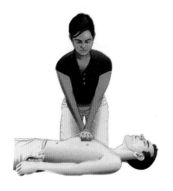

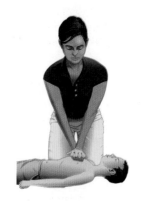

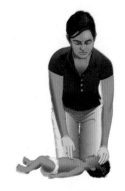

| **Adult** | **Child** | **Infant** |
|---|---|---|
| About age 12 years or older | Between the ages of 1 and 12 years | Younger than 1 year |

## Hand Position

| | | |
|---|---|---|
| Two hands in center of chest | Two hands in center of chest | Two fingers on center of chest, just below the nipple line |

## Chest Compressions

| | | |
|---|---|---|
| Compress **at least 2** inches | Compress **about 2** inches | Compress **about 1½** inches |
| Rate: 100–120 compressions/min | Rate: 100–120 compressions/min | Rate: 100–120 compressions/min |

## Rescue Breaths

| | | |
|---|---|---|
| Tilt head to **past-neutral position**; pinch nose shut and form seal over mouth | Tilt head to **slightly past-neutral position**; pinch nose shut and form seal over mouth | Tilt head to **neutral position**; form seal over mouth and nose |

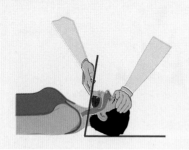

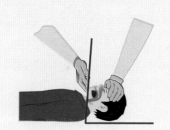

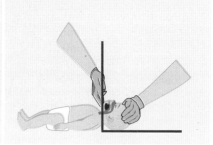

## Sets

| | | |
|---|---|---|
| 30 chest compressions and 2 rescue breaths | 30 chest compressions and 2 rescue breaths | 30 chest compressions and 2 rescue breaths |

your arms straight, push down at least 2 inches, and then let the chest completely return to its normal position. Push hard and push fast! You want to go at a rate of 100–120 compressions per minute. As you give compressions, count out loud up to 30. Maintain a smooth, steady down-and-up rhythm and do not pause between compressions.

- **Give a set of 2 rescue breaths.** Once you have given 30 compressions, give 2 rescue breaths. First, open the airway using the **head-tilt/chin-lift maneuver**. Place one of your hands on the person's forehead and two fingers of your other hand on the bony part of the person's chin. Tilt the person's head back and lift the chin. For an adult, tilt the head to a past-neutral position (see Table 3-1). If possible, use a CPR breathing barrier when you are giving rescue breaths, but do not delay rescue breaths to find a breathing barrier or learn how to use it. Pinch the person's nose shut. Take a normal breath, make a complete seal over the person's mouth with your mouth, and blow into the person's mouth to give the first rescue breath. Take another breath, make a seal, and give the second rescue breath. Each rescue breath should last about 1 second and make the person's chest rise. After you finish giving 2 rescue breaths, return to giving compressions as quickly as possible. The process of giving 2 rescue breaths and getting back to compressions should take less than 10 seconds. Never give more than 2 rescue breaths per set. Table 3-2 describes how to troubleshoot special situations when giving rescue breaths.

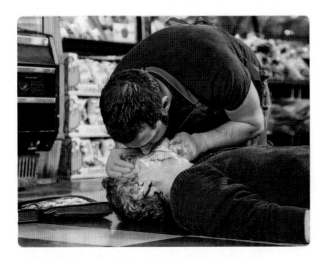

Once you begin CPR, continue giving sets of 30 chest compressions and 2 rescue breaths until:

- You notice an obvious sign of life, such as movement. (If the person shows an obvious sign of life, stop CPR, place the person in the recovery position and continue to monitor the person's condition until EMS personnel take over.)

- An AED is ready to use and no other trained responders are available to assist you with the AED.

**THE PROS KNOW.**

———

Counting out loud as you give compressions can help you to keep a steady, even rhythm. For compressions 1 through 12, say "one and two and three and four and five and six and..." up to 12. When you get to 13, just say the number: "thirteen, fourteen, fifteen, sixteen..." up to 30. Push down as you say the number and come up as you say "and" (or the second syllable of the number). This will help you to keep a steady, even rhythm.

**THE PROS KNOW.**

———

Incorrect technique or body position can cause your arms and shoulders to tire quickly when you are giving compressions. Use the weight of your upper body to compress the chest, not your arm muscles. Avoid rocking back and forth, because rocking makes your compressions less effective and wastes your energy. Also avoid leaning on the chest, because leaning prevents the chest from returning to its normal position after each compression, limiting the amount of blood that can return to the heart.

**THE PROS KNOW.**

———

When giving rescue breaths, keep the person's head tilted back and avoid taking too large of a breath or blowing too forcefully. Failing to keep the person's head tilted back, taking too large of a breath, or blowing too forcefully can force air into the person's stomach instead of into his or her lungs, which can make the person vomit and cause other complications. Remember: Keep the head tilted back, take a normal breath and blow just enough to make the chest rise.

# TABLE 3-2 Special Situations: Rescue Breathing

| Special Situation | Solution |
|---|---|
| **The breaths do not make the chest rise.** 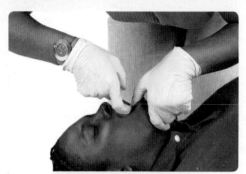 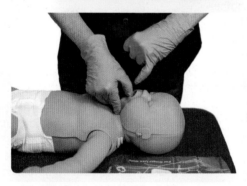 | Never give more than 2 rescue breaths per set. If the first rescue breath does not cause the chest to rise, retilt the head to ensure that the airway is properly opened and ensure that the person's nose and mouth are properly sealed before giving the second rescue breath. If the second breath does not make the chest rise, an object may be blocking the person's airway. Give CPR with one modification: after each set of compressions and before giving rescue breaths, open the mouth, look for an object in the person's mouth, and if you see it, remove it. |
| **The person vomits or there is fluid in the mouth.** 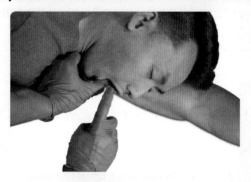 | Roll the person onto his or her side and clear the mouth of fluid using a gloved finger or a piece of gauze. Then roll the person onto his or her back and resume giving care. |
| **You are unable to form a tight seal over the person's mouth (e.g., due to an injury).** 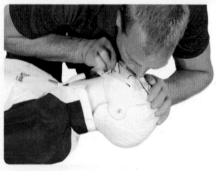 | Use mouth-to-nose breathing instead. With the person's head tilted back, close the person's mouth by pushing on the person's chin. Make a complete seal over the person's nose with your mouth and blow in for 1 second to make the chest rise. |

*(Continued)*

| Special Situation | Solution |
|---|---|
| The person has a **tracheostomy** or "stoma," a surgically created opening in the front of the neck that opens into the trachea (windpipe) to form an alternate route for breathing when the upper airway is blocked or damaged. | Use mouth-to-stoma breathing instead. Expose the person's neck down to the breastbone and remove anything covering the stoma (e.g., a filter or stoma cover). Wipe away any secretions from the stoma. Make a complete seal over the person's stoma or tracheostomy tube with your mouth and blow in for 1 second to make the chest rise.<br><br>■ If the chest does not rise, the tracheostomy tube may be blocked. Remove the inner tube and try rescue breaths again.<br><br>■ If you hear or feel air escaping from the person's mouth or nose, the person is a partial neck breather (i.e., there is still a connection between the trachea and the upper airway, and although the person breathes mainly through the stoma, he or she is also able to breathe to some extent through the mouth and nose). Seal the person's mouth and nose with your hand or a tight-fitting mask so that air does not escape out of the mouth or nose when you give rescue breaths into the stoma. |
| ■ You have performed approximately 2 minutes of CPR (5 sets of 30:2) and another trained responder is available to take over compressions. Giving chest compressions correctly is physically tiring. If more than one responder is available and trained in CPR, the responders should switch responsibility for compressions every 2 minutes, or whenever the responder giving compressions indicates that he or she is tiring. Switching responsibility for giving chest compressions frequently reduces responder fatigue, which improves the quality of chest compressions and leads to a better chance of survival for the person. | ■ You have performed approximately 2 minutes of CPR (5 sets of 30:2), you are alone and caring for a child, and you need to call 9-1-1 or the designated emergency number.<br><br>■ EMS personnel take over.<br><br>■ You are alone and too tired to continue.<br><br>■ The scene becomes unsafe. |

## Giving CPR to a Child

Giving CPR to a child is very similar to giving CPR to an adult. However, in a child, you open the airway by tilting the head to a slightly past-neutral position, rather than to a past-neutral position (see Table 3-1). Rather than compressing the chest to a depth of *at least* 2 inches as you would for an adult, you compress the chest to a depth of *about* 2 inches for a child. Also, for a small child, you may only need to give compressions with one hand, instead of two.

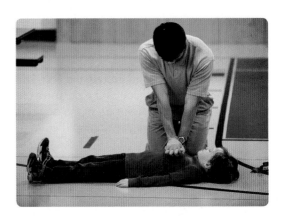

## Giving CPR to an Infant

The general principles of giving CPR to an infant are the same as they are for children and adults. However, because the infant's body is smaller, you will position your hands differently to deliver compressions. Place the pads of two fingers on the center of the infant's chest, just below the nipple line. If you feel the notch at the end of the infant's breastbone, move your fingers slightly toward the infant's head. Place your other hand on the infant's forehead. Give compressions by using the pads of your fingers to compress the chest about 1½ inches.

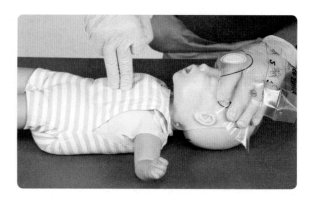

When you give rescue breaths, open the airway by tilting the head to a neutral position (see Table 3-1). Instead of pinching the nose shut and covering the mouth with your mouth, cover the infant's nose and mouth with your mouth to form a seal.

# Using an AED

Different types of AEDs are available, but all are similar to operate and use visual displays, voice prompts or both to guide the responder. If your place of employment has an AED on site, know where it is located, how to operate it and how to maintain it (Box 3-3). Also take note of the location of AEDs in public places that you frequent, such as shopping centers, airports, recreation centers and sports arenas.

When a person is in cardiac arrest, use an AED as soon as possible. Skill Sheet 3-4 describes how to use an AED step by step. Environmental and person-specific considerations for safe and effective AED use are given in Box 3-4.

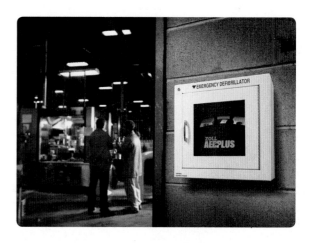

## Using an AED on an Adult

To use an AED, first turn the device on. Remove or cut away clothing and undergarments to expose the person's chest. If the person's chest is wet, dry it using a towel or gauze pad. Dry skin helps the AED pads to stick properly. Do not use an alcohol wipe to dry the skin because alcohol is flammable. Next, apply the AED pads. Peel the backing off the pads as directed, one at a time, to expose the adhesive. Place one pad on the upper right side of the person's chest and the other pad on the lower left side of the person's chest below the armpit, pressing firmly to adhere (Figure 3-7). Plug the connector cable into the AED (if necessary) and follow the device's directions. Most AEDs will begin to analyze the heart rhythm automatically, but some may require you to push an "analyze" button to start this process. No one should touch the person while the AED is analyzing the heart rhythm because this could result in a faulty reading. Next, the AED

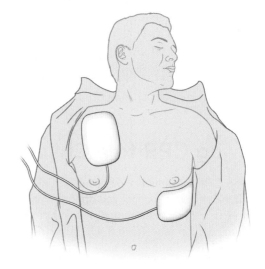

**Figure 3-7.** Place one AED pad on the upper right side of the chest and the other on the lower left side of the chest, below the armpit.

will tell you to push the "shock" button if a shock is advised. Again, avoid touching the person, because anyone who is touching the person while the device is delivering a shock is at risk for receiving a shock as well. After a shock is delivered (or if the AED determines that no shock is necessary), immediately resume CPR, starting with compressions. The AED will continue to check the heart rhythm every 2 minutes. Listen for prompts from the AED and continue giving CPR and using the AED until you notice an obvious sign of life or EMS personnel arrive. If you notice an obvious sign of life, stop CPR but leave the AED turned on and the pads in place on the person's chest, and continue to follow the AED's prompts.

## Using an AED on a Child or Infant

The procedure for using an AED on a child or infant is the same as the procedure for using an AED on an adult. Some AEDs come with pediatric AED pads that are smaller and designed specifically to analyze a child's heart rhythm and deliver a lower level of energy. These pads should be used on children up to 8 years of age or weighing less than 55 pounds. Other AEDs have a key or switch that configures the AED for use on a child up to 8 years of age or weighing less than 55 pounds. If pediatric AED pads are not available or the

## Box 3-3. AED Maintenance

AEDs require minimal maintenance, but it is important to check them regularly according to the manufacturer's instructions or your employer's policy to ensure that they are in good working order and ready for use whenever they are needed.

■ Familiarize yourself with the owner's manual and follow the manufacturer's instructions for maintaining the equipment.

■ Familiarize yourself with the method the AED uses to indicate the status of the device. Many AEDs have a status indicator that displays a symbol or illuminates to indicate that the AED is in proper working order and ready to respond. The status indicator may also display symbols indicating that routine maintenance (e.g., a battery change) is needed or that a problem with the device has been detected. Some AEDs have a warning indicator that will illuminate or beep if the AED is not in proper working order and ready to respond.

■ Check to make sure the battery is properly installed and within its expiration date.

■ Make sure AED pads are adequately stocked, stored in a sealed package, and within their expiration date.

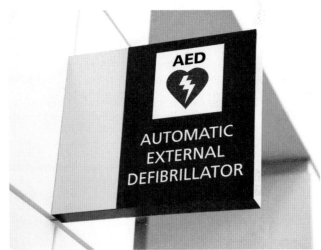

■ After using the AED, make sure that all supplies are restocked and that the device is in proper working order.

■ If at any time the AED fails to work properly or warning indicators illuminate, take the AED out of service and contact the manufacturer or the appropriate person at your place of employment, according to your employer's policy. You may need to return the AED to the manufacturer for service. If the AED stops working during an emergency, continue giving CPR until EMS personnel take over.

AED does not have a pediatric setting, it is safe to use adult AED pads and adult levels of energy on a child or infant. (Note that the opposite is not true—you should not use pediatric AED pads or the pediatric setting on an adult because the shock delivered will not be sufficient if the person is older than 8 years or weighs more than 55 pounds.)

Just as when you are using an AED on an adult, apply the AED pads to the child's bare, dry chest, placing one pad on the upper right chest and the other pad on the lower left side of the chest below the armpit. If you cannot position the pads this way without them touching (as in the case of an infant or a small child), position one pad in the middle of the chest and the other pad on the back between the shoulder blades (Figure 3-8). Then follow the standard procedure for using an AED.

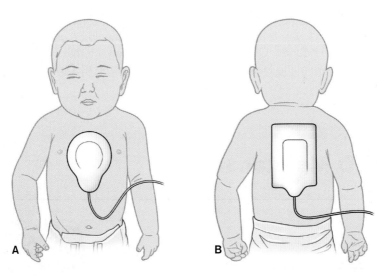

**Figure 3-8.** If the person is too small to place both AED pads on the front of the chest without them touching, place one on the middle of the chest (A) and the other between the shoulder blades (B).

---

# Box 3-4. **Considerations for Safe and Effective AED Use**

## Environmental Considerations

- **Flammable or combustible materials.** Do not use an AED around flammable or combustible materials, such as gasoline or free-flowing oxygen.

- **Metal surfaces.** It is safe to use an AED when the person is lying on a metal surface, as long as appropriate precautions are taken. Do not allow the AED pads to contact the metal surface, and ensure that no one is touching the person when the shock is delivered.

- **Water.** If the person is in water, remove him or her from the water before using the AED. Once you have removed the person from the water, be sure there are no puddles of water around you, the person or the AED.

- **Inclement weather.** It is safe to use AEDs in all weather conditions, including rain and snow. Provide a dry environment if possible (for example, by sheltering the person with umbrellas), but do not delay defibrillation to do so. Remove wet clothing and wipe the person's chest dry before placing the AED pads. Avoid getting the AED or AED pads wet.

*(Continued)*

# Person-Specific Considerations

- **Pregnancy.** It is safe to use an AED on a woman who is pregnant.

- **Pacemakers and implantable cardioverter-defibrillators (ICDs).** A person who has a known arrhythmia (irregular heartbeat) may have a pacemaker or an ICD. These are small devices that are surgically implanted under the skin to automatically prevent or correct an irregular heartbeat. You may be able to see or feel the outline of the pacemaker or ICD in the area below the person's collarbone, or the person may wear medical identification indicating that he or she has a pacemaker or ICD. If the implanted device is visible or you know that the person has a pacemaker or ICD, adjust pad placement as necessary to avoid placing the AED pads directly over the device because doing so may interfere with the delivery of the shock. However, if you are not sure whether the person has an implanted device, place the pads as you normally would.

- **Transdermal medication patches.** Some types of medications, including nitroglycerin (used to relieve chest pain caused by cardiovascular disease) and smoking-cessation medications, are delivered through patches applied to the skin. Remove any medication patches that you see before applying AED pads and using an AED. Wear gloves to prevent absorption of the drug through your own skin.

- **Chest hair.** Time is critical in a cardiac arrest situation and chest hair rarely interferes with pad adhesion, so in most cases, you should proceed as you normally would—attach the AED pads, pressing firmly to attach them. However, if the person has a great deal of thick chest hair and it seems like the chest hair could interfere with pad-to-skin contact, quickly shave the areas where the pads will be placed and then attach the pads.

- **Jewelry and body piercings.** You do not need to remove the person's jewelry or body piercings before using an AED, but you should avoid placing the AED pads directly over any metallic jewelry or piercings. Adjust pad placement if necessary.

# Working as a Team

Remember, when you are giving CPR, you want to give high-quality compressions at the appropriate depth and rate. You also want to minimize interruptions to chest compressions. If you are the only trained responder at the scene, you will begin to tire as you give CPR, and the quality of your compressions will diminish. You will also need to stop CPR to ready the AED for use when it arrives, which means that during that time, there is no oxygenated blood moving through the person's body.

Working as a team can lead to a better chance of survival for the person in cardiac arrest, by reducing responder fatigue and minimizing interruptions to chest compressions. Trained responders can share the responsibility for giving compressions, switching off every 2 minutes, which reduces fatigue and leads to better-quality compressions. Having two or more trained responders at the scene also minimizes interruptions to chest compressions when the AED arrives.

When two or more responders trained in CPR and using an AED are at the scene, all should identify themselves as being trained. The first responder should begin CPR while the second responder calls 9-1-1 or the designated emergency number, obtains the AED and readies the AED for use by turning the device on, applying the pads to the person's chest and plugging in the connector cable, if necessary (Figure 3-9). The first responder should not pause CPR until the device is ready to analyze the person's heart rhythm and the second responder tells everyone to stand clear. While the AED is analyzing, the responders should switch roles so that the second responder can take over giving chest compressions. The responder who is taking over compressions should hover with his or hands positioned just above the person's chest so that he or she can immediately start compressions as soon as the AED prompts that a shock was delivered or that no shock was advised. The responders then switch roles every time the AED analyzes the person's heart rhythm, which occurs every 2 minutes.

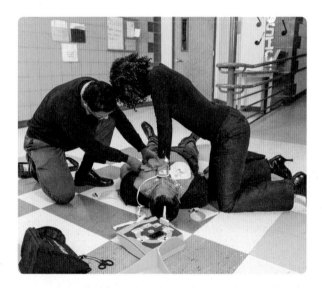 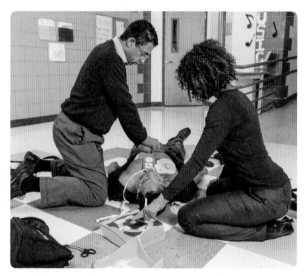

**Figure 3-9.** Working as a team can lead to a better chance of survival for the person in cardiac arrest.

# Giving CPR to an Adult

1. Verify that the person is unresponsive and not breathing.

   ■ Shout to get the person's attention, using the person's name if you know it. If the person does not respond, tap the person's shoulder and shout again while checking for normal breathing.

   ■ If the person does not respond and is not breathing or only gasping, continue to step 2.

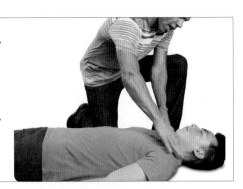

2. Place the person on his or her back on a firm, flat surface. Kneel beside the person.

3. Give **30** chest compressions.

   ■ Place the heel of one hand in the center of the person's chest, with your other hand on top. Position your body so that your shoulders are directly over your hands.

   ■ Keeping your arms straight, push down at least 2 inches, and then let the chest return to its normal position.

   ■ Push hard and push fast! Give compressions at a rate of 100–120 compressions per minute.

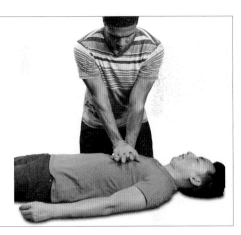

4. Give **2** rescue breaths.

   ■ Place the breathing barrier over the person's nose and mouth.

   ■ Open the airway. (Put one hand on the forehead and two fingers on the bony part of the chin and tilt the head back to a past-neutral position.)

   ■ Pinch the nose shut and make a complete seal over the person's mouth with your mouth.

   ■ Take a normal breath and blow into the person's mouth for about 1 second, looking to see that the chest rises.

   ■ Take another breath, make a seal, then give the second rescue breath.

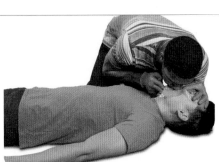

**Note:** *If the first rescue breath does not cause the chest to rise, retilt the head and ensure a proper seal before giving the second rescue breath. If the second breath does not make the chest rise, an object may be blocking the airway. After the next set of chest compressions and before attempting rescue breaths, open the mouth, look for an object and, if seen, remove it using a finger sweep. Continue to check the person's mouth for an object after each set of compressions until the rescue breaths go in.*

*(Continued)*

5.  Continue giving sets of **30** chest compressions and **2** rescue breaths until:

■   You notice an obvious sign of life.

■   An AED is ready to use and no other trained responders are available to assist you with the AED.

■   You have performed approximately 2 minutes of CPR (5 sets of 30:2) and another trained responder is available to take over compressions.

■   EMS personnel take over.

■   You are alone and too tired to continue.

■   The scene becomes unsafe.

# Giving CPR to a Child

1. Verify that the child is unresponsive and not breathing.

   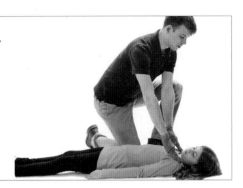

   ■ Shout to get the child's attention, using the child's name if you know it. If the child does not respond, tap the child's shoulder and shout again while checking for normal breathing.

   ■ If the child does not respond and is not breathing or only gasping, continue to step 2.

2. Place the child on his or her back on a firm, flat surface. Kneel beside the child.

3. Give **30 chest compressions.**

   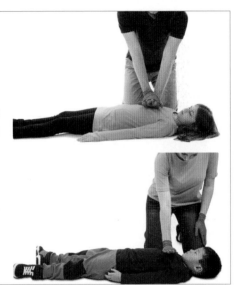

   ■ Place the heel of one hand in the center of the child's chest, with your other hand on top. Position your body so that your shoulders are directly over your hands. (Alternatively, in a small child, you can use a one-handed CPR technique: place the heel of one hand in the center of the child's chest.)

   ■ Keeping your arms straight, push down about 2 inches, and then let the chest return to its normal position.

   ■ Push hard and push fast! Give compressions at a rate of 100–120 compressions per minute.

4. Give **2 rescue breaths.**

   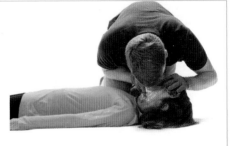

   ■ Place the breathing barrier over the child's nose and mouth.

   ■ Open the airway. (Put one hand on the forehead and two fingers on the bony part of the chin and tilt the head back to a slightly past-neutral position.)

   ■ Pinch the nose shut and make a complete seal over the child's mouth with your mouth.

   ■ Take a normal breath and blow into the child's mouth for about 1 second, looking to see that the chest rises.

   ■ Take another breath, make a seal, then give the second rescue breath.

*(Continued)*

# Giving CPR to a Child continued

**Note:** *If the first rescue breath does not cause the chest to rise, retilt the head and ensure a proper seal before giving the second rescue breath. If the second breath does not make the chest rise, an object may be blocking the airway. After the next set of chest compressions and before attempting rescue breaths, open the mouth, look for an object and, if seen, remove it using a finger sweep. Continue to check the child's mouth for an object after each set of compressions until the rescue breaths go in.*

5. Continue giving sets of **30** chest compressions and **2** rescue breaths until:

   ■ You notice an obvious sign of life.

   ■ An AED is ready to use and no other trained responders are available to assist you with the AED.

   ■ You have performed approximately 2 minutes of CPR (5 sets of 30:2) and another trained responder is available to take over compressions.

   ■ You have performed approximately 2 minutes of CPR (5 sets of 30:2), you are alone and caring for a child, and you need to call 9-1-1 or the designated emergency number.

   ■ EMS personnel take over.

   ■ You are alone and too tired to continue.

   ■ The scene becomes unsafe.

# Giving CPR to an Infant

1. Verify that the infant is unresponsive and not breathing.

   - Shout to get the infant's attention, using the infant's name if you know it. If the infant does not respond, tap the bottom of the infant's foot and shout again while checking for normal breathing.

   - If the infant does not respond and is not breathing or only gasping, continue to step 2.

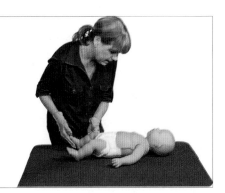

2. Place the infant on his or her back on a firm, flat surface. Stand or kneel next to the infant.

3. Give **30** chest compressions.

   - Place one hand on the infant's forehead.

   - Place the pad of two fingers on the center of the infant's chest, just below the nipple line.

   - Compress the chest about 1½ inches, and then let the chest return to its normal position.

   - Push hard and push fast! Give compressions at a rate of 100–120 compressions per minute.

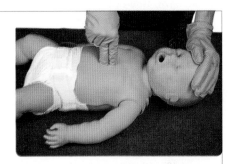

4. Give **2** rescue breaths.

   - Place the breathing barrier over the infant's nose and mouth.

   - Open the airway. (Put one hand on the forehead and two fingers on the bony part of the chin and tilt the head back to a neutral position.)

   - Make a complete seal over the infant's nose and mouth with your mouth.

   - Take a normal breath and blow into the infant's nose and mouth for about 1 second, looking to see that the chest rises.

   - Take another breath, make a seal, then give the second rescue breath.

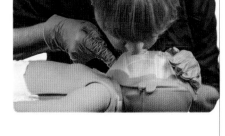

**Note:** *If the first rescue breath does not cause the chest to rise, retilt the head and ensure a proper seal before giving the second rescue breath. If the second breath does not make the chest rise, an object may be blocking the airway. After the next set of chest compressions and before attempting rescue breaths, open the mouth, look for an object and, if seen,*

*(Continued)*

# Giving CPR to an Infant continued

*remove it using a finger sweep. Continue to check the infant's mouth for an object after each set of compressions until the rescue breaths go in.*

5.  Continue giving sets of **30** chest compressions and **2** rescue breaths until:

    ■   You notice an obvious sign of life.

    ■   An AED is ready to use and no other trained responders are available to assist you with the AED.

    ■   You have performed approximately 2 minutes of CPR (5 sets of 30:2) and another trained responder is available to take over compressions.

    ■   You have performed approximately 2 minutes of CPR (5 sets of 30:2), you are alone and caring for an infant, and you need to call 9-1-1 or the designated emergency number.

    ■   EMS personnel take over.

    ■   You are too tired to continue.

    ■   The scene becomes unsafe.

# Using an AED

**Note:** *Do not use pediatric AED pads on an adult or on a child older than 8 years or weighing more than 55 pounds. However, adult AED pads can be used on a child younger than 8 years or weighing less than 55 pounds if pediatric AED pads are not available.*

1. Turn on the AED and follow the voice prompts.

2. Remove all clothing covering the chest and, if necessary, wipe the chest dry.

3. Place the pads.

   - Place one pad on the upper right side of the chest and the other on the lower left side of the chest below the armpit.

   - If the pads may touch (e.g., on an infant or small child), place one pad in the middle of the chest and the other pad on the back, between the shoulder blades.

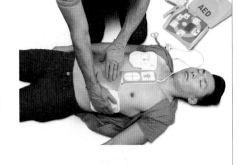

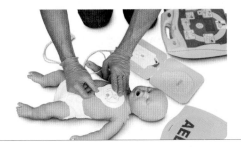
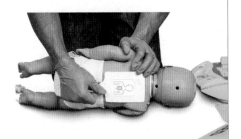

4. Plug the connector cable into the AED, if necessary.

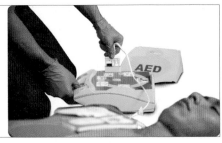

*(Continued)*

# Using an AED continued

5. Prepare to let the AED analyze the heart's rhythm.

   - Make sure no one, including you, is touching the person. Say, "EVERYONE CLEAR!" in a loud, commanding voice.

   - If the AED tells you to, push the "analyze" button to start this process.

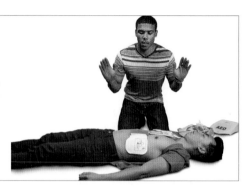

6. Deliver a shock, if the AED determines one is needed.

   - Make sure no one, including you, is touching the person. Say, "EVERYONE CLEAR!" in a loud, commanding voice.

   - Push the "shock" button to deliver the shock.

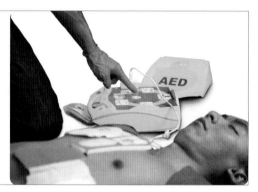

7. After the AED delivers the shock, or if no shock is advised:

   - Immediately begin CPR, starting with compressions. Continue giving CPR (about 2 minutes, or 5 sets of 30:2) until prompted by the AED.

   - Continue giving CPR and following the AED's prompts until you see an obvious sign of life or EMS personnel arrive.

# CHOKING

**C**hoking is especially common in young children, but a person of any age can choke. Choking occurs when the airway becomes either partially or completely blocked by a foreign object, such as a piece of food or a small toy; by swelling in the mouth or throat; or by fluids, such as vomit or blood. A person who is choking can quickly become unresponsive and die, so it is important to act quickly.

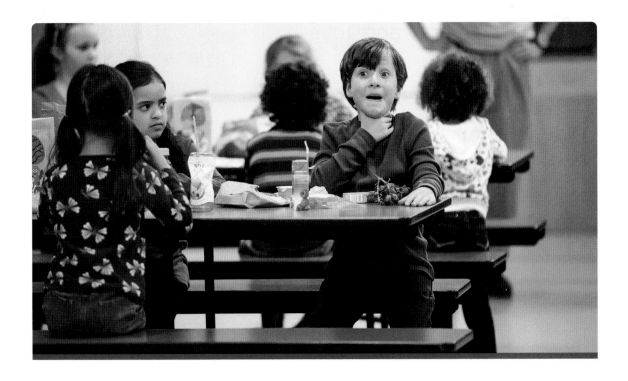

# Risk Factors for Choking

Certain behaviors can put a person at risk for choking, such as talking or laughing with the mouth full or eating too fast. Medical conditions (such as a neurological or muscular condition that affects the person's ability to chew, swallow or both) can increase risk for choking. So can dental problems or poorly fitting dentures that affect the person's ability to chew food properly.

Children younger than 5 years are at particularly high risk for choking (Box 4-1). Infants and toddlers explore by putting things in their mouths and can easily choke on them. Even some common foods can be choking hazards in young children. For example, a young child can choke on small foods (such as nuts and seeds);

---

## Box 4-1. **Choking Hazards**

In children younger than 4 years, the following foods, household objects and toys may be choking hazards:

### Foods

- Nuts and seeds
- Hot dogs and sausages
- Chunks of meat or cheese
- Chunks of fruit (such as apples) and whole grapes
- Raw vegetables (such as carrots and celery)
- Popcorn
- Peanut butter

- Hard, gooey or sticky candy (such as peppermint candies, fruit strips, marshmallows, gummy bears and chewing gum)
- Large foods that break easily into small pieces (such as teething biscuits and cookies)

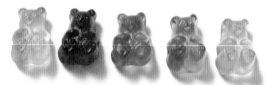

### Household Objects and Toys

- Plastic bags, broken or uninflated balloons, and disposable gloves (the thin material can block the airway)
- Coins
- Buttons
- Small "button" batteries (found inside watches, car key fobs, singing greeting cards, hearing aids and other electronics)
- Magnets
- Marbles
- Beads
- Pebbles
- Pen or marker caps

- Safety pins and hairpins
- Jewelry
- Baby powder
- Vitamins
- Items from the trash (such as eggshells or the pull tabs from soda cans)
- Toys meant for older children, which may be small or have small parts*

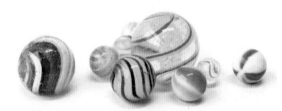

*For infants and toddlers, no toy should be smaller than 1¾ inches in diameter. If you can fit the toy through a toilet paper tube, then it is too small and not safe for a young child.

round, firm foods (such as grapes, hot dogs and hard candies); and sticky foods (such as peanut butter). This is because young children do not have the skills needed to chew these foods thoroughly, so they often try to just swallow them whole. Laughing, talking or running with the mouth full can also lead to choking.

# Signs and Symptoms of Choking

A person who is choking typically has a panicked, confused or surprised facial expression. Some people may place one or both hands on their throat. The person may cough (either forcefully or weakly), or he or she may not be able to cough at all. You may hear high-pitched squeaking noises as the person tries to breathe, or nothing at all. If the airway is totally blocked, the person will not be able to speak, cry or cough. The person's skin may initially appear flushed (red), but will become pale or bluish in color as the body is deprived of oxygen.

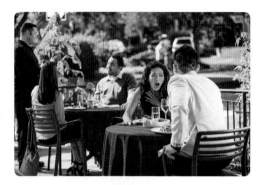

# First Aid for Choking

If you are with a person who starts to choke, first ask the person if he or she is choking, or check to see if an infant is crying or making other noises. If the person can speak or cry and is coughing forcefully, encourage him or her to keep coughing. A person who is getting enough air to speak, cry or cough forcefully is getting enough air to breathe. But be prepared to act if the person's condition changes.

If the person is making high-pitched noises or coughing weakly, or if the person is unable to speak or cry, the airway is blocked and the person will soon become unresponsive unless the airway is cleared. Have someone call 9-1-1 or the designated emergency number immediately while you begin to give first aid for choking.

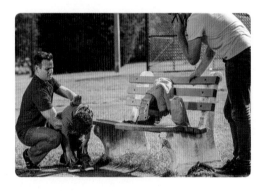

## Caring for an Adult or Child Who Is Choking

When an adult or child is choking, give a combination of 5 **back blows** (blows between the shoulder blades) followed by 5 **abdominal thrusts** (inward and upward thrusts just above the navel) (Figure 4-1). The goal of giving back blows and abdominal thrusts is to force the object out of the airway, allowing the person to breathe.

- **Back blows.** To give back blows, position yourself to the side and slightly behind the person. For a child, you may need to kneel. Place one arm diagonally across the person's chest (to provide support) and bend the person forward at the waist so that the person's upper body is as close to parallel to the ground as possible. Firmly strike the person between the shoulder blades with the heel of your other hand. Each back blow should be separate from the others.

- **Abdominal thrusts.** To give abdominal thrusts, stand behind the person, with one foot in front

of the other for balance and stability. If possible, place your front foot between the person's feet. Wrap your arms around the person's waist. Alternatively, if the person is a child, you can kneel behind the child, wrapping your arms around the child's waist. Find the person's navel by placing one finger on the person's navel, and the adjacent finger above the first. Make a fist with your other hand and place the thumb side just above your fingers. Cover your fist with your other hand and give quick, inward and upward thrusts into the person's abdomen. Each abdominal thrust should be separate from the others.

Continue giving sets of back blows and abdominal thrusts until the person can cough forcefully, speak, cry, or breathe, or the person becomes unresponsive. After the choking incident is over, even if the person seems fine, he or she should still be evaluated by a healthcare provider to make sure there is no damage to the airway or other internal injuries.

For step-by-step instructions on giving first aid to an adult or child who is choking, see Skill Sheets 4-1 and 4-2. Table 4-1 describes how to troubleshoot special situations when an adult or child is choking.

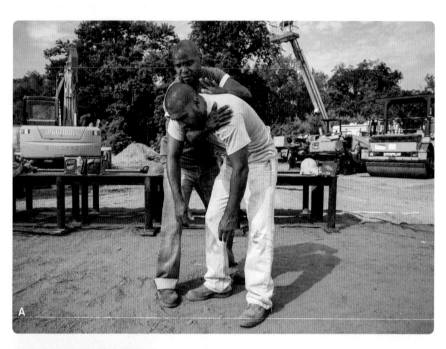

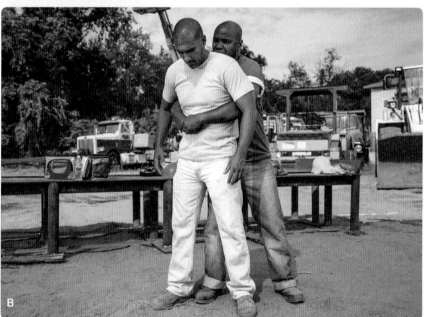

**Figure 4-1.** Use a combination of back blows (A) and abdominal thrusts (B) when an adult or child is choking.

# TABLE 4-1 Special Situations: Choking in an Adult or Child

| Special Situation | Solution |
|---|---|
| **The person is too large for you to wrap your arms around to give abdominal thrusts.** 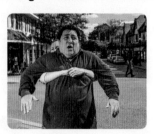 | Give chest thrusts instead of abdominal thrusts. To give chest thrusts, position yourself behind the person as you would for abdominal thrusts. Place the thumb side of your fist against the center of the person's breastbone. Then cover your fist with your other hand and pull straight back, giving a quick, inward thrust into the person's chest. |
| **The person is obviously pregnant or known to be pregnant.** 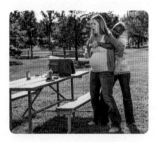 | Give chest thrusts instead of abdominal thrusts. |
| **The person is in a wheelchair.** 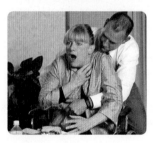 | Give abdominal thrusts in the same way that you would for a person who is standing. It may be necessary to kneel behind the wheelchair. If features of the wheelchair make it difficult to give abdominal thrusts, give chest thrusts instead. |
| **You are alone and choking.** 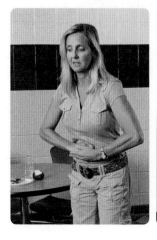 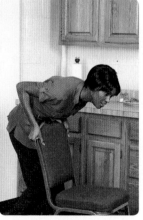 | Call 9-1-1 or the designated emergency number using a landline or a GPS-enabled mobile phone. Even if you are not able to speak, the open line will cause the dispatcher to send help. Give yourself abdominal thrusts, using your hands, just as if you were giving abdominal thrusts to another person. Alternatively, bend over and press your abdomen against any firm object, such as the back of a chair or a railing. Do not bend over anything with a sharp edge or corner that might hurt you, and be careful when leaning on a railing that is elevated. |

# Caring for an Infant Who Is Choking

When an infant is choking, give a combination of 5 back blows followed by 5 chest thrusts (instead of abdominal thrusts) (Figure 4-2). You can sit, kneel or stand to give first aid care to a choking infant, as long as you are able to support the infant on your thigh with the infant's head lower than his or her chest. If the infant is large or your hands are small, you may find it easiest to sit or kneel.

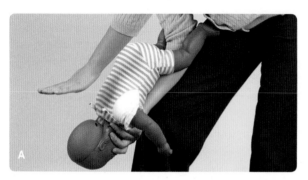
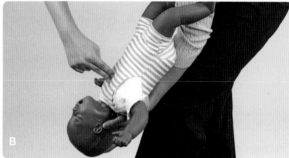

**Figure 4-2.** Use a combination of back blows (A) and chest thrusts (B) when an infant is choking.

- **Back blows.** First, get the infant into position for back blows. Place your forearm along the infant's back, cradling the back of the infant's head with your hand. Place your other forearm along the infant's front, supporting the infant's jaw with your thumb and fingers. (Be careful not to cover the infant's mouth with your hand while you are supporting the infant's jaw.) Turn the infant over so that he or she is face-down along your forearm. Lower your arm onto your thigh so that the infant's head is lower than his or her chest. Continue to support the infant's jaw with the thumb and fingers of one hand while you firmly strike the infant between the shoulder blades with the heel of your other hand. Keep your fingers up to avoid hitting the infant's head or neck. Each back blow should be separate from the others.

- **Chest thrusts.** Next, place one hand along the infant's back, cradling the back of the infant's head with your hand. While continuing to support the infant's jaw with the thumb and fingers of your other hand, support the infant between your forearms and turn the infant over so that he or she is face-up along your forearm. Lower your arm onto your thigh so that the infant's head is lower than his or her chest. Place the pads of two fingers in the center of the infant's chest, on the breastbone just below the nipple line. Press down about 1 ½ inches and then let the chest return to its normal position, keeping your fingers in contact with the breastbone. Each chest thrust should be separate from the others.

Continue sets of 5 back blows and 5 chest thrusts until the infant can cough forcefully, cry or breathe, or the infant becomes unresponsive. After the choking incident is over, even if the infant seems fine, he or she should still be evaluated by a healthcare provider to make sure there is no damage to the airway or other internal injuries.

For step-by-step instructions on giving first aid to an infant who is choking, see Skill Sheet 4-3.

# If the Person Becomes Unresponsive

If a person who is choking becomes unresponsive, carefully lower him or her to the ground and, if you are trained, begin CPR, starting with chest compressions. After each set of chest compressions and before attempting rescue breaths, open the person's mouth and look for the object. If you see an object in the person's mouth, remove it using your finger (Figure 4-3). Never put your finger in the person's mouth unless you actually see the object. If you cannot see the object and you put your finger in the person's mouth, you might accidentally push the object deeper into the person's throat.

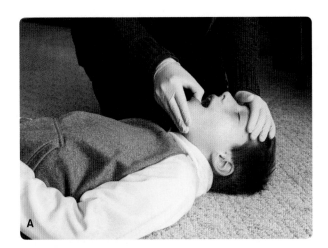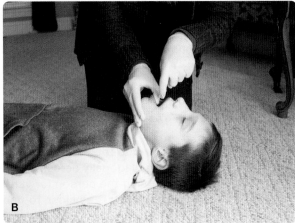

**Figure 4-3.** If the person becomes unresponsive, look for the object in the person's mouth (A), and if you see it, use a finger sweep to remove it (B).

# Caring for an Adult Who Is Choking

1. Verify that the person is choking by asking the person to speak to you.

   - **If the person is able to speak to you or is coughing forcefully:** Encourage the person to keep coughing, but be prepared to give first aid for choking if the person's condition changes.

   - **If the person is unable to speak to you or is coughing weakly:** Send someone to call 9-1-1 or the designated emergency number and to obtain an AED and first aid kit. Continue to step 2 after obtaining consent.

2. Give **5** back blows.

   - Position yourself to the side and slightly behind the person. Place one arm diagonally across the person's chest (to provide support) and bend the person forward at the waist so that the person's upper body is as close to parallel to the ground as possible.

   - Firmly strike the person between the shoulder blades with the heel of your hand.

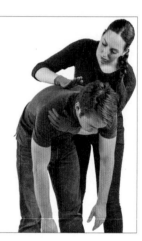

3. Give **5** abdominal thrusts.

   - Have the person stand up straight. Stand behind the person with one foot in front of the other for balance and wrap your arms around the person's waist.

   - Using two fingers of one hand, find the person's navel. With your other hand, make a fist and place the thumb side against the person's stomach, right above your fingers.

   - Cover the fist with your other hand.

   - Pull inward and upward to give an abdominal thrust.

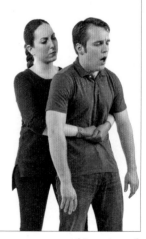

*(Continued)*

4. Continue giving sets of **5** back blows and **5** abdominal thrusts until:

- The person can cough forcefully, speak, cry or breathe.

- The person becomes unresponsive.

**Note:** *If the person becomes unresponsive, gently lower him or her to the floor and begin CPR if you are trained, starting with compressions. After each set of compressions and before attempting rescue breaths, open the person's mouth, look for the object and remove it if seen. Never put your finger in the person's mouth unless you actually see the object.*

# Caring for a Child Who Is Choking

1. Verify that the child is choking by asking the child to speak to you.

   - **If the child is able to speak to you or is coughing forcefully:** Encourage the child to keep coughing, but be prepared to give first aid for choking if the child's condition changes.

   - **If the child is unable to speak to you or is coughing weakly:** Send someone to call 9-1-1 or the designated emergency number and to obtain an AED and first aid kit. Continue to step 2 after obtaining consent.

2. Give **5** back blows.

   - Position yourself to the side and slightly behind the child. Place one arm diagonally across the child's chest (to provide support) and bend the child forward at the waist so that the child's upper body is as close to parallel to the ground as possible. Depending on the child's size, you may need to kneel.

   - Firmly strike the child between the shoulder blades with the heel of your hand.

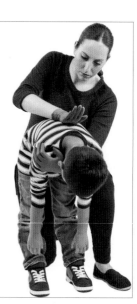

3. Give **5** abdominal thrusts.

   - Have the child stand up straight. Stand behind the child with one foot in front of the other for balance (or kneel) and wrap your arms around the child's waist.

   - Using two fingers of one hand, find the child's navel. With your other hand, make a fist and place the thumb side against the child's stomach, right above your fingers.

   - Cover the fist with your other hand.

   - Pull inward and upward to give an abdominal thrust.

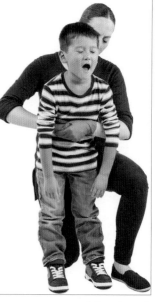

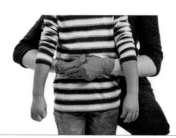

*(Continued)*

4. Continue giving sets of **5** back blows and **5** abdominal thrusts until:

  ■ The child can cough forcefully, speak, cry or breathe.

  ■ The child becomes unresponsive.

**Note:** *If the child becomes unresponsive, gently lower him or her to the floor and begin CPR if you are trained, starting with compressions. After each set of compressions and before attempting rescue breaths, open the child's mouth, look for the object and remove it if seen. Never put your finger in the child's mouth unless you actually see the object.*

# Caring for an Infant Who Is Choking

1. Verify that the infant is choking by checking to see if the infant is crying or coughing forcefully.

   - **If the infant is crying or coughing forcefully:** Allow the infant to keep coughing, but be prepared to give first aid for choking if the infant's condition changes.

   - **If the infant is unable to cry or is coughing weakly:** Send someone to call 9-1-1 or the designated emergency number and to obtain an AED and first aid kit. Continue to step 2 after obtaining consent.

2. Position the infant.

   - Place your forearm along the infant's back, cradling the back of the infant's head with your hand.

   - Place your other forearm along the infant's front, supporting the infant's jaw with your thumb and fingers.

   - Turn the infant over so that he or she is face-down along your forearm.

   - Lower your arm onto your thigh so that the infant's head is lower than his or her chest.

   **Note:** *Always support the infant's head, neck and back while giving back blows and chest thrusts.*

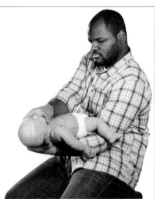

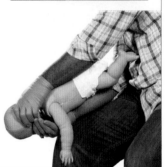

3. Give 5 back blows.

   - Firmly strike the infant between the shoulder blades with the heel of your hand. Keep your fingers up to avoid hitting the infant's head or neck.

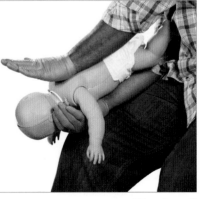

*(Continued)*

4. Reposition the infant.

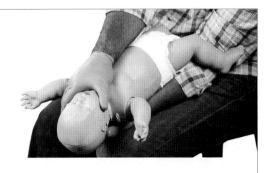

- Place one hand along the infant's back, cradling the back of the infant's head with your hand.

- While continuing to support the infant's jaw with the thumb and fingers of your other hand, support the infant between your forearms and turn the infant over so that he or she is face-up along your forearm.

- Lower your arm onto your other thigh so that the infant's head is lower than his or her chest.

5. Give **5 chest thrusts**.

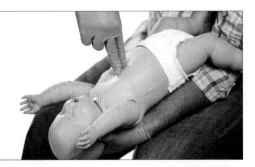

- Place the pads of two fingers in the center of the infant's chest on the breastbone, just below the nipple line.

- Press down about 1½ inches and then let the chest return to its normal position.

6. Continue giving sets of **5 back blows** and **5 chest thrusts** until:

- The infant can cough forcefully, cry or breathe.

- The infant becomes unresponsive.

**Note:** *If the infant becomes unresponsive, lower him or her to a firm, flat surface and begin CPR if you are trained, starting with compressions. After each set of compressions and before attempting rescue breaths, open the infant's mouth, look for the object and remove it if seen. Never put your finger in the infant's mouth unless you actually see the object.*

# PART 3

First Aid for
Common
Illnesses and
Injuries

# 5

# SUDDEN ILLNESS

Illness often strikes with little to no warning, at work, at school, at home or while we are out having fun. When a person becomes suddenly ill, you can help by providing appropriate first aid care; summoning help, if needed; and keeping the person comfortable until help arrives.

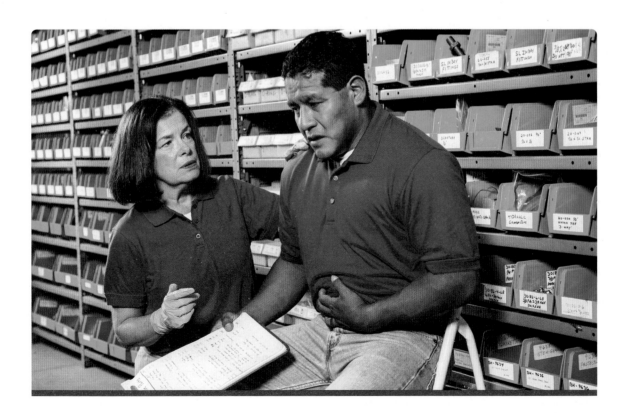

# General Approach to Sudden Illness

An **acute illness** is an illness that strikes suddenly and usually only lasts for a short period of time. A **chronic illness** is an illness that a person lives with on an ongoing basis and that often requires continuous treatment to manage. When a person becomes suddenly ill, it may be the result of an acute illness, or it may be an acute flare-up of a chronic condition.

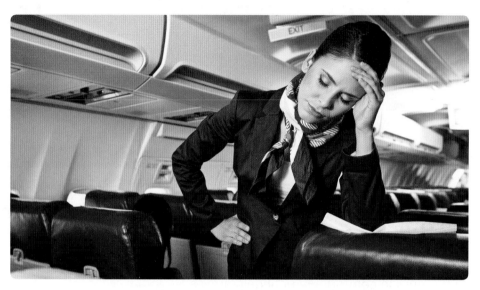

## Signs and Symptoms of Sudden Illness

The signs and symptoms of sudden illness vary widely, depending on the cause of the illness. The person may have:

- Trouble breathing.

- Pain, such as chest pain, abdominal pain or a headache.

- Changes in level of consciousness, such as being confused or unaware of one's surroundings, or becoming unresponsive.

- Light-headedness or dizziness.

- Nausea, vomiting, diarrhea or stomach cramps.

- A fever.

- Pale or very flushed skin, which may be excessively sweaty or dry, or excessively hot or cold.

- Problems seeing or speaking (e.g., blurred vision or slurred speech).

- Numbness, weakness or paralysis.

- Seizures.

**THE PROS KNOW.**

___

Sarah Smith
Type I Diabetes
ICE:555-555-5555

Be sure to look for a medical identification tag or digital medical identification on the person's phone when you are checking the person. It may offer a valuable clue as to the cause of the person's sudden illness.

To gain a better understanding of the situation, interview the person (or bystanders, if necessary) using SAMPLE, and then check the person from head-to-toe (see Chapter 2). Signs and symptoms like trouble breathing, pain that is persistent or severe, problems seeing or speaking, problems feeling or moving, seizures or unresponsiveness require a call to 9-1-1 or the designated emergency number. If you are unsure about the severity of the illness, it is better to call for help early than to wait for the illness to progress.

# First Aid Care for Sudden Illness

Fortunately, you do not need to know exactly what is wrong to provide appropriate first aid care. If your initial check of the person reveals any life-threatening conditions (see Chapter 1, Box 1-5), make sure that someone calls 9-1-1 or the designated emergency number right away, and then provide care according to the signs and symptoms that you find and your level of training. Follow the same general guidelines as you would for any emergency:

- Do no further harm.
- Monitor the person's breathing and level of consciousness.
- Help the person rest in the most comfortable position.
- Keep the person from getting chilled or overheated.
- Reassure the person that you will help and that EMS personnel have been called (if appropriate).
- Give care consistent with your knowledge and training as needed, and continue to watch for changes in the person's condition.

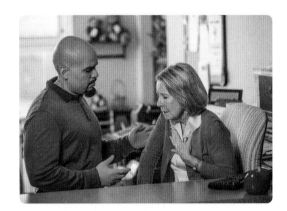

# Respiratory Distress

**Respiratory distress**, or difficulty breathing, is evidenced by signs and symptoms such as shortness of breath, gasping for breath, **hyperventilation** (breathing that is faster and shallower than normal), or breathing that is uncomfortable or painful. Respiratory distress can lead to **respiratory arrest** (absence of breathing).

## Causes of Respiratory Distress

A number of different conditions can cause respiratory distress, including acute flare-ups of chronic respiratory conditions such as asthma or chronic obstructive pulmonary disease (COPD); lung and respiratory tract infections (such as pneumonia or bronchitis); severe allergic reactions (anaphylaxis); heart conditions (such as a heart attack or heart failure); trauma; poisoning; drug overdose; electrocution; and mental health conditions (such as panic disorder).

## Signs and Symptoms of Respiratory Distress

A person who is experiencing respiratory distress is, understandably, often very frightened. The person may feel like he or she cannot get enough air and may gasp for breath. Because the person is struggling to breathe, speaking in complete sentences may be difficult. You might hear wheezing, gurgling or high-pitched noises as the person tries to breathe. You may also notice that the person's breathing is unusually slow or fast, unusually deep or shallow, or irregular. The person's skin may feel moist or cool, and it may be pale, ashen (gray), bluish or flushed. Lack of oxygen can make the person feel dizzy or light-headed.

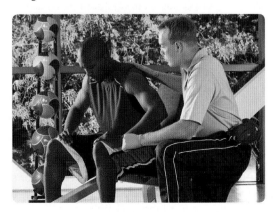

# First Aid Care for Respiratory Distress

When a person is experiencing a breathing emergency, it is important to act at once. In some breathing emergencies, the oxygen supply to the body is greatly reduced, whereas in others the oxygen supply is cut off entirely. If breathing stops or is restricted long enough, the person will become unresponsive, the heart will stop beating and body systems will quickly fail. Recognizing that a person is having trouble breathing and providing appropriate first aid care can save the person's life.

You usually can identify a breathing problem by watching and listening to the person's breathing and by asking the person how he or she feels. If a person is having trouble breathing, do not wait to see if the person's condition improves. Call 9-1-1 or the designated emergency number and provide appropriate first aid care until help arrives:

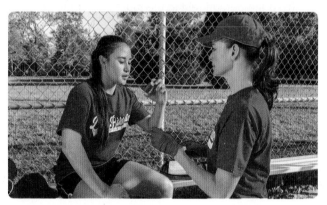

- If you know the cause of the respiratory distress (for example, an asthma attack or anaphylaxis) and the person carries medication used for the emergency treatment of the condition, offer to help the person take his or her medication.

- Encourage the person to sit down and lean forward. Many people find that this position helps to make breathing easier. Providing reassurance can reduce anxiety, which may also help to make breathing easier.

- If the person is responsive, gather additional information by interviewing the person and performing a head-to-toe check. Remember that a person having breathing problems may find it difficult to talk. Try phrasing your questions as "yes" or "no" questions so the person can nod or shake his or her head in response instead of making the effort to speak. You may also be able to ask bystanders what they know about the person's condition.

- Be prepared to give CPR and use an AED if the person becomes unresponsive and you are trained in these skills.

# Asthma

Many people have **asthma**, a chronic illness in which certain substances or conditions, called **triggers**, cause inflammation and narrowing of the airways, making breathing difficult. Common triggers include exercise, temperature extremes, allergies, air pollution, strong odors (such as perfume, cologne and scented cleaning products), respiratory infections, and stress or anxiety. The trigger causes inflammation and swelling, which causes the opening of the airways to become smaller and makes it harder for air to move in and out of the lungs. People who have asthma usually know what can trigger an attack and take measures to avoid these triggers.

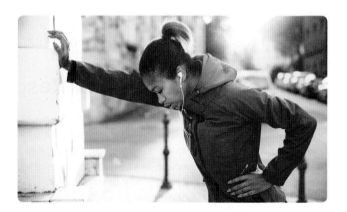

A person who has been diagnosed with asthma may take two forms of medication. **Long-term control medications** are taken regularly, whether or not signs and symptoms of asthma are present. These medications help prevent asthma attacks by reducing inflammation and swelling and making the airways less sensitive to triggers. **Quick-relief (rescue) medications** are taken when the person is experiencing an acute asthma attack. These medications work quickly to relax the muscles that tighten around the airways, opening the airways right away so that the person can breathe more easily. Both long-term control medications and quick-relief (rescue) medications may be given through an inhaler, a nebulizer (Box 5-1) or orally.

---

## Box 5-1. **Asthma Inhalers and Nebulizers**

The most common way to take long-term control and quick-relief (rescue) medications is by inhaling them. Inhalation allows the medication to reach the airways faster and work quickly. There also are fewer side effects. Medications are inhaled using a metered dose inhaler (MDI), a dry powder inhaler (DPI) or a small-volume nebulizer.

### Metered Dose Inhalers (MDIs)

An MDI delivers a measured dose of medication in mist form directly into the person's lungs. The person gently presses down the top of the inhaler. This causes a small amount of pressurized gas to push the medication out quickly. Sometimes a spacer (or chamber) is used to make it easier for the person to use the inhaler correctly. The medication goes into the spacer, and then the person inhales the medication through the mouthpiece on the spacer. For children, a spacer may be used with a face mask instead of a mouthpiece.

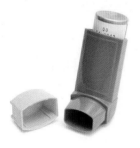

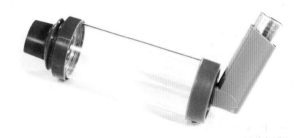

### Dry Powder Inhalers (DPIs)

A DPI delivers a measured dose of medicine in a dry powder form directly into the person's lungs. Instead of pressing down on the top of the device to dispense the medication, the person breathes in quickly to activate the DPI and dispense the medication. Some people have difficulty using DPIs because they require the user to take in a quick, strong breath.

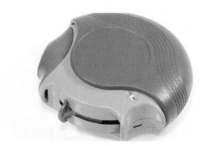

### Small-Volume Nebulizers

Small-volume nebulizers convert liquid medication into a mist, which is delivered over several minutes. Nebulizers are especially helpful when the person is unable to take deep breaths, for children younger than 5 years and for older adults. They also are used for people who have trouble using inhalers and for those with severe asthma.

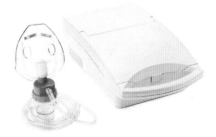

# Signs and Symptoms of an Asthma Attack

Even when a person takes steps to manage his or her asthma by avoiding triggers and taking prescribed long-term control medications, he or she may still experience asthma attacks occasionally. Signs and symptoms of an asthma attack include:

- Wheezing or coughing.

- Rapid, shallow breathing (or trouble breathing).

- Sweating.

- Being unable to talk without stopping for a breath in between every few words.

- Feelings of tightness in the chest or being unable to get enough air into the lungs.

- Anxiety and fear.

## First Aid Care for an Asthma Attack

An asthma attack can become life threatening because it affects the person's ability to breathe. If the person has an **asthma action plan** (a written plan that the person develops with his or her healthcare provider that details daily management of the condition as well as how to handle an asthma attack), help the person to follow that plan. Encourage the person to use his or her prescribed quick-relief (rescue) medication, assisting if needed and if state or local regulations allow. (Skill Sheet 5-1 provides step-by-step instructions for helping a person to use an asthma inhaler.) If you have not already done so, call 9-1-1 or the designated emergency number if the person's breathing does not improve after taking the quick-relief (rescue) medication or if the person becomes unresponsive. Stay with the person and monitor his or her condition until the person is able to breathe normally or help arrives.

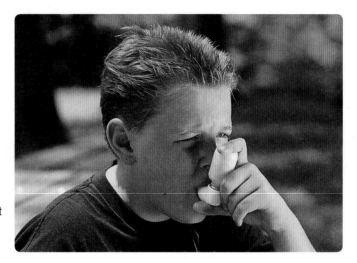

# Allergic Reactions and Anaphylaxis

Our immune systems help to keep us healthy by fighting off harmful pathogens that can cause disease. But sometimes our immune systems overreact and try to fight off ordinary things that are not usually harmful, like certain foods, grass or pet dander (tiny flakes of skin that animals shed). A person can have an allergy to almost anything. Common allergens (allergy triggers) include venomous insect stings, certain foods (like peanuts, tree nuts, shellfish, milk, eggs, soy and wheat), animal dander, plant pollen, certain medications (like penicillin and sulfa drugs) and latex.

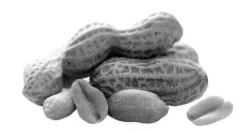

# Signs and Symptoms of Allergic Reactions and Anaphylaxis

An allergic reaction can range from mild to very severe. A person who is having a mild to moderate allergic reaction may develop a skin rash, a stuffy nose, or red, watery eyes. The skin or area of the body that came in contact with the allergen usually swells and turns red.

A person who is having a severe, life-threatening allergic reaction (called **anaphylaxis**) may develop one or more of the following signs and symptoms within seconds or minutes of coming into contact with the allergen:

- Trouble breathing

- Swelling of the face, neck, tongue or lips

- A feeling of tightness in the chest or throat

- Skin reactions (such as hives, itchiness or flushing)

- Stomach cramps, nausea, vomiting or diarrhea

- Dizziness

- Loss of consciousness

- Signs and symptoms of shock (such as excessive thirst; skin that feels cool or moist and looks pale or bluish; an altered level of consciousness; and a rapid, weak heartbeat)

To determine if a person is having a severe, life-threatening allergic reaction (anaphylaxis), look at the situation as well as the person's signs and symptoms (Table 5-1).

## TABLE 5-1 How Do I Know If It Is Anaphylaxis?

| Situation | Look For: |
|---|---|
| You do not know if the person has been exposed to an allergen. | <ul><li>Any skin reaction (such as hives, itchiness or flushing) **OR**</li><li>Swelling of the face, neck, tongue or lips</li></ul>**PLUS**<ul><li>Trouble breathing **OR**</li><li>Signs and symptoms of shock</li></ul> |
| You think the person may have been exposed to an allergen. | Any **TWO** of the following:<ul><li>Any skin reaction</li><li>Swelling of the face, neck, tongue or lips</li><li>Trouble breathing</li><li>Signs and symptoms of shock</li><li>Nausea, vomiting, cramping or diarrhea</li></ul> |
| You know that the person has been exposed to an allergen. | <ul><li>Trouble breathing</li></ul>**OR**<ul><li>Signs and symptoms of shock</li></ul> |

# First Aid Care for Allergic Reactions and Anaphylaxis

If you know that the person has had a severe allergic reaction before, and the person is having trouble breathing or is showing signs and symptoms of anaphylaxis, have someone call 9-1-1 or the designated emergency number immediately. If the person carries medication (e.g., epinephrine) used for the emergency treatment of anaphylaxis, offer to help the person use the medication. If you are alone, help the person administer the medication and then call 9-1-1 or the designated emergency number. While you wait for help to arrive, make sure the person is sitting in a comfortable position, or have the person lie down if he or she is showing signs of shock.

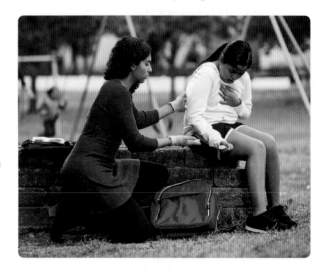

## Epinephrine

**Epinephrine** is a drug that slows or stops the effects of anaphylaxis. If a person is known to have an allergy that could lead to anaphylaxis, he or she may carry an **epinephrine auto injector** (a syringe system, available by prescription only, that contains a single dose of epinephrine). Devices are available containing different doses because the dose of epinephrine is based on weight (0.15 mg for children weighing between 33 and 66 pounds, and 0.3 mg for children and adults weighing more than 66 pounds). Many healthcare providers advise that people with a known history of anaphylaxis carry an anaphylaxis kit containing at least two doses of epinephrine (two auto injectors) with them at all times. This is because more than one dose may be needed to stop the anaphylactic reaction. Have the person administer a second dose only if emergency responders are delayed and the person is still having signs and symptoms of anaphylaxis 5 to 10 minutes after administering the first dose.

It is important to act fast when a person is having an anaphylactic reaction because difficulty breathing and shock are both life-threatening conditions. If the person is unable to self-administer the medication, you may need to help. You may assist a person with using an epinephrine auto injector when the person has a previous diagnosis of anaphylaxis and has been prescribed an epinephrine auto injector; the person is having signs and symptoms of anaphylaxis; the person requests your help using an auto injector; and your state laws

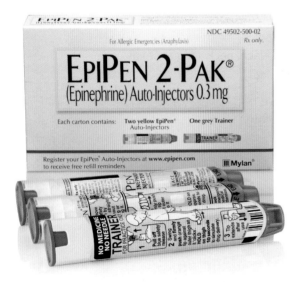

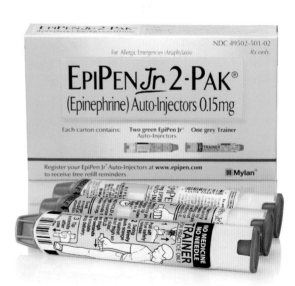

permit giving assistance. Where state and local laws allow, some organizations (such as schools) keep a stock epinephrine auto injector for designated staff members who have received the proper training to use in an anaphylaxis emergency. If you are using a stock epinephrine auto injector, follow your organization's emergency action plan, which may include verifying that the person is showing signs and symptoms of anaphylaxis, ensuring that the person has been prescribed epinephrine in the past, and making sure to use a device containing the correct dose based on the person's weight.

Different brands of epinephrine auto injectors are available, but all work in a similar fashion (and some have audio prompts to guide the user). The device is activated by pushing it against the mid-outer thigh. Once activated, the device injects the epinephrine into the thigh muscle. The device must be held in place for the recommended amount of time (5 to 10 seconds, depending on the device) to deliver the medication. Some medication may still remain in the auto injector even after the injection is complete. After removing the auto injector, massage the injection site for several seconds (or have the person massage the injection site). Handle the used device carefully to prevent accidental needlestick injuries. Place the device in a rigid container, and then give the container to EMS personnel for proper disposal. For step-by-step instructions on helping a person to use an epinephrine auto injector, see Skill Sheet 5-2.

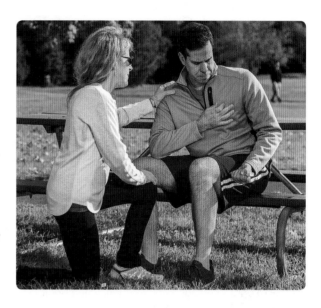

## Antihistamines

The person's healthcare provider may recommend that the person carry an antihistamine in his or her anaphylaxis kit, in addition to epinephrine. An **antihistamine** is a medication that counteracts the effects of histamine, a chemical released by the body during an allergic reaction. Antihistamines are supplied as pills, capsules or liquids and are taken by mouth. The person should take the antihistamine according to the medication label and his or her healthcare provider's instructions.

# Diabetic Emergencies

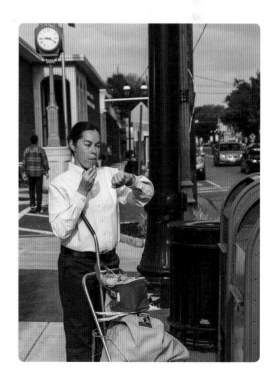

**Diabetes** is a chronic condition characterized by the body's inability to process glucose (sugar) in the bloodstream. An organ called the pancreas secretes **insulin**, a hormone that causes glucose to be moved from the bloodstream into the cells, where it is used for energy. In a person with diabetes, either the pancreas fails to make enough insulin or the body's cells are unable to respond to insulin. Either situation causes glucose levels in the bloodstream to increase.

A person with diabetes may manage the condition with insulin injections or oral medications. Diet and exercise also play an important role. To keep blood glucose levels within an acceptable range, food intake, exercise and medication must be balanced. A person with diabetes must follow a well-balanced diet, with limited sweets and fats. The timing of meals and snacks relative to exercise and medication is important as well.

If food intake, exercise and medication are not in balance, the person may experience a diabetic emergency.

- **Hypoglycemia** (excessively low blood glucose levels) can result if a person misses a meal or snack, eats too little food, exercises more than usual, vomits or takes too much medication.

- **Hyperglycemia** (excessively high blood glucose levels) can result if a person eats too much food, takes too little medication, exercises less than usual or experiences physical or emotional stress.

## Signs and Symptoms of Diabetic Emergencies

A person who is having a diabetic emergency will seem generally ill. He or she may feel dizzy or shaky, have a headache, or have cool, clammy skin. The person's behavior may change (for example, he or she may become irritable, aggressive or argumentative). If the person is experiencing hyperglycemia, his or her breath may have a fruity or sweet odor. Severe hypoglycemia or hyperglycemia can result in confusion, seizures or loss of consciousness and may be life threatening.

## First Aid Care for Diabetic Emergencies

Call 9-1-1 or the designated emergency number if the person is unresponsive, not fully awake or having a seizure. While you wait for help to arrive, provide appropriate care. For example, if the person is not fully awake, interview bystanders and conduct a head-to-toe check, then put the person in the recovery position. Make sure the person's airway is clear of vomit and monitor the person's breathing until help arrives. If the person is having a seizure, take steps to keep the person safe while you let the seizure run its course.

If the person is known to have diabetes and thinks he or she is having a diabetic emergency, you may be able to help the person by giving him or her some form of sugar. Only offer the person sugar by mouth if the person is responsive, able to answer your questions and able to swallow. Some people may be responsive but not fully awake and therefore not able to safely swallow; in this case, do not attempt to give the person sugar by mouth. Instead, call 9-1-1 or the designated emergency number. You should also call 9-1-1 or the designated emergency number if you are not able to immediately obtain an acceptable form of sugar. Acceptable forms of sugar include:

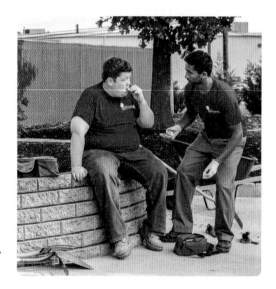

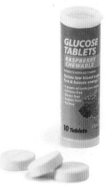

- Glucose tablets.

- Candies that can be chewed.

- Fruit juice.

- Fruit strips.

- Regular (non-diet) soda.

- Milk.

- A spoonful of sugar mixed into a glass of water.

If it is safe for the person to have sugar by mouth, give 15 to 20 grams of sugar. Check the label on packaged products to determine how much of the package's contents to give. Even if the person is experiencing hyperglycemia (too much glucose in the bloodstream), giving the person 15 to 20 grams of sugar will not cause additional harm. If possible, have the person check his or her blood glucose level. If the person is not feeling better in about 10 to 15 minutes, call 9-1-1 or the designated emergency number.

Some people with diabetes may have a prescribed glucagon kit that they carry with them to use in case of a severe hypoglycemic emergency. Glucagon is a hormone that stimulates the liver to release glucose into the bloodstream. The glucagon kit is only used when the person is unresponsive or has lost the ability to swallow. Those who spend a significant amount of time with the person (for example, family members, teachers, coaches or co-workers) may receive additional training to learn how to administer a glucagon injection.

# Seizures

A **seizure** is the result of abnormal electrical activity in the brain, leading to temporary and involuntary changes in body movement, function, sensation, awareness or behavior. Seizures can have many different causes. One common cause is **epilepsy**, a chronic seizure disorder that can often be controlled with medication. Other causes of seizure include fever, infection, diabetic emergencies, heat stroke and injuries to the brain tissue.

## Signs and Symptoms of Seizures

There are different types of seizures. One common type of seizure is called a grand mal seizure. A person having a grand mal seizure loses consciousness and has **convulsions** (uncontrolled body movements caused by contraction of the muscles). Another common type of seizure is called an absence seizure. The person experiences a brief, sudden lapse of consciousness, causing the person to momentarily become very quiet and have a blank stare. A person with epilepsy may experience an **aura** (an unusual sensation or feeling) before the onset of the seizure. If the person recognizes the aura, he or she may have time to tell someone what is happening and sit down before the seizure occurs.

## First Aid Care for Seizures

Although a seizure can be frightening to see, it is easy to care for a person who is having a seizure. Most seizures only last a few minutes, and the person usually recovers fully without any complications. If the person is known to have occasional seizures, it may not be necessary to call 9-1-1 or the designated emergency number. However, under some circumstances, you should call 9-1-1 or the designated emergency number when a person is having a seizure. Call for help if:

- The seizure lasts more than 5 minutes, or the person has multiple seizures in a row.

- The person was injured as a result of the seizure.

- The person is unresponsive and not breathing or only gasping after the seizure.

- The person is pregnant or has diabetes.

- The person is a young child or infant and the seizure was brought on by a high fever.

- The person is elderly.

- This is the person's first seizure, or the cause of the seizure is unknown.

- The seizure took place in the water.

When a person is having a seizure, do not try to hold the person down or stop the seizure from happening. Just let the seizure run its course and take steps to protect the person from injury. Move furniture or other objects that could cause injury out of the way. The person may be drowsy and disoriented for as long as 20 minutes after the seizure is over. Check the person for responsiveness and normal breathing. If the person is responsive and breathing normally but not yet fully awake, check the person from head to toe for injuries and then place the person in the recovery position. Stay with the person until he or she is fully recovered and aware of his or her surroundings, or until emergency responders arrive. If the person is not responsive and not breathing or only gasping after the seizure, begin CPR immediately and use an AED as soon as possible, if you are trained in these skills.

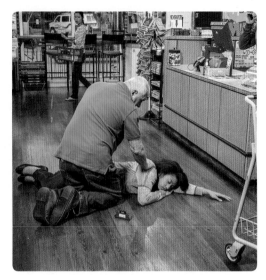

**Myth-Information.** *Myth: Put something between the teeth of person who is having a seizure to prevent the person from biting or swallowing his or her tongue.* This practice is unsafe and unnecessary. It is impossible to swallow one's own tongue. And although the person may bite down on his or her tongue, causing it to bleed, this is a minor problem compared with the problems that can be caused by attempting to put an object in the mouth of a person who is having a seizure. You could chip a tooth or knock a tooth loose, putting the person at risk for choking. The person may also bite down with enough force to break the object and then choke on a piece of the object. Additionally, attempting to place an object in the person's mouth puts you at risk for getting bitten.

# Fainting

If a person suddenly loses consciousness and then "comes to" after about a minute, he or she may simply have fainted. Fainting is caused by a sudden decrease in blood flow to the brain. Usually the cause of fainting is not serious. For example, being dehydrated (not having enough fluid in the body), being too hot, being in a crowded room or feeling intense emotion can cause a person to faint. After the person faints, the head is at the same level as the heart. This helps blood flow return to the brain and the person quickly recovers.

## Signs and Symptoms of Fainting

A person who is about to faint often becomes pale, begins to sweat and may feel weak or dizzy. The person may sense that he or she is about to faint and may attempt to sit down to prevent a fall.

## First Aid Care for Fainting

The person may faint before you even know what is happening, but sometimes it is possible to prevent a fainting spell by having the person sit down with his or her head near his or her knees, or lie down flat on his or her back. If the person does faint, check the person for responsiveness and normal breathing. If the person responds and is breathing normally, check the person from head to toe for injuries that might have happened as a result of the fall. If there are no injuries, place the person in the recovery position and loosen any tight clothing. Call 9-1-1 or the designated emergency number if you find any injuries or have any concerns about the person's condition. Although the cause of fainting is not usually serious, the person should still follow up with his or her healthcare provider. If the person does not respond and is not breathing or is only gasping, begin CPR immediately and use an AED as soon as possible, if you are trained in these skills.

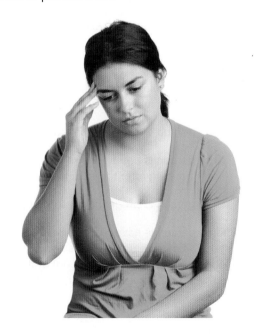

# Stroke

A **stroke** occurs when blood flow to part of the brain is interrupted by a blood clot, resulting in the death of brain cells. A stroke can also be caused by bleeding into the brain tissue. Strokes can cause permanent brain damage, but with quick action, sometimes the damage can be stopped or reversed. Although strokes are most common in older adults, a person of any age, even a child, can have a stroke.

Some people experience **transient ischemic attacks (TIAs)**, or "mini-strokes." TIAs cause signs and symptoms similar to those of a stroke, but the signs and symptoms go away after a short period of time. A person who has had a TIA is at very high risk for having a stroke in the near future. In fact, more than 10 percent of people who have a TIA will have a stroke within 3 months, with half of these strokes happening within 48 hours of the TIA. For this reason, whenever a person experiences signs and symptoms of stroke, even if the signs and symptoms seem to go away, the person should seek immediate medical attention.

## Signs and Symptoms of Stroke

The signs and symptoms of stroke can vary from person to person. A person who is having a stroke may suddenly develop one or more of the following signs and symptoms:

- Trouble with speech and language, including slurring of words, being unable to form words or being unable to understand what others are saying

- Drooling or difficulty swallowing

- Drooping of the features on one side of the face (for example, the eyelid and the corner of the mouth)

- Trouble seeing in one or both eyes

- Weakness

- Paralysis or numbness of the face, arms or legs, especially on one side of the body

- A sudden, severe headache

- Dizziness or loss of balance

- Confusion

- Loss of consciousness

The "FAST" check (Figure 5-1) is a quick way of checking for signs and symptoms of stroke.

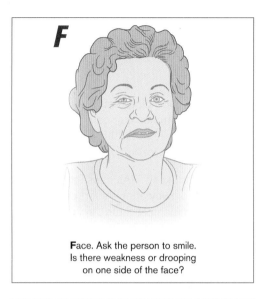

Face. Ask the person to smile. Is there weakness or drooping on one side of the face?

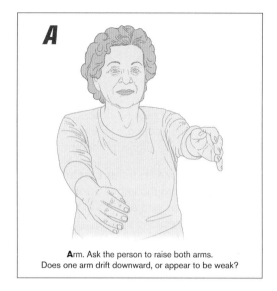

Arm. Ask the person to raise both arms. Does one arm drift downward, or appear to be weak?

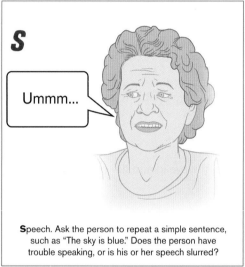

Ummm...

Speech. Ask the person to repeat a simple sentence, such as "The sky is blue." Does the person have trouble speaking, or is his or her speech slurred?

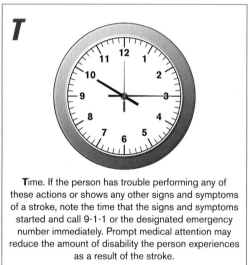

Time. If the person has trouble performing any of these actions or shows any other signs and symptoms of a stroke, note the time that the signs and symptoms started and call 9-1-1 or the designated emergency number immediately. Prompt medical attention may reduce the amount of disability the person experiences as a result of the stroke.

**Figure 5-1.** The FAST check for stroke.

# First Aid Care for Stroke

If you think that a person is having (or has had) a stroke, call 9-1-1 or the designated emergency number immediately. Note when the signs and symptoms first started (or, if you do not know when the signs and symptoms started, note the last time the person was known to be well). This is important information to give to EMS personnel because some of the medications used to treat stroke are only effective within a certain time frame after the onset of signs and symptoms. Stay with the person and provide reassurance until help arrives. If the person is responsive but not fully awake, or if the person is drooling or having trouble swallowing, put the person in the recovery position and monitor the person's condition until EMS personnel arrive.

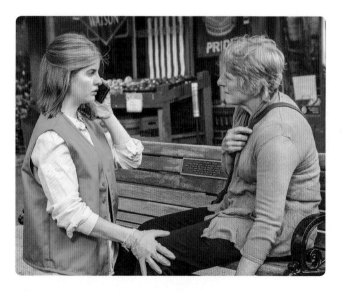

# Assisting with an Asthma Inhaler

**Note**: *The instructions for assisting a person with an asthma inhaler found on this skill sheet should not be substituted for those given by the manufacturer and the person's healthcare provider. Read and follow all instructions printed on the inhaler prior to assisting the person with administering the medication, and consult the person's asthma control plan.*

1. Help the person to sit up and lean slightly forward to make breathing easier.

2. Verify with the person that the medication is for "quick relief" or "acute attacks." Also check the expiration date on the inhaler.

   ▪ If the medication is not for "quick relief" or "acute attacks," do not use it.

   ▪ If the medication is expired, do not use it.

3. Shake the inhaler.

4. Remove the mouthpiece cover. If the person uses a spacer, attach it to the mouthpiece.

   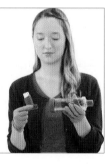

5. Ask the person to breathe out as much as possible through the mouth.

*(Continued)*

# Assisting with an Asthma Inhaler continued

6. Help the person to take the medication.

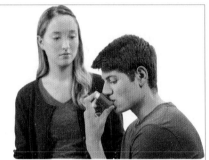

- **No spacer.** Position the mouthpiece of the inhaler according to the method the person uses. Some people may close their lips tightly around the mouthpiece of the inhaler. Others may hold the mouthpiece an inch or two away from the mouth. Have the person take a long, slow breath (about 3 to 5 seconds) while pressing down on the top of the canister. Then have the person hold his or her breath for a count of 10.

- **Spacer.** Have the person close his or her lips tightly around the spacer and push the button on the top of the canister to release the medication into the spacer. Have the person take a long, slow breath (about 3 to 5 seconds), and then hold the breath for a count of 10.

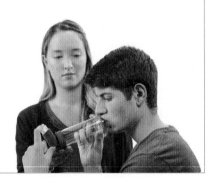

- **Spacer with mask.** Position the mask over the person's nose and mouth. Have the person push the button on the top of the canister to release the medication into the spacer. Have the person breathe in and out normally about 5 or 6 times.

7. Note the time. The person's breathing should improve within 5 to 15 minutes. More than one dose of medication may be needed to stop the asthma attack. The label will tell you how long to wait between doses.

- If the person's breathing does not improve or the person becomes unresponsive, call 9-1-1 or the designated emergency number.

# Assisting with an Epinephrine Auto Injector

**Note**: *The instructions for assisting a person with an epinephrine auto injector found on this skill sheet should not be substituted for those given by the manufacturer and the person's healthcare provider.*

**Note:** *You may assist a person with using an epinephrine auto injector when the person has a previous diagnosis of anaphylaxis and has been prescribed an epinephrine auto injector; the person is having signs and symptoms of anaphylaxis; the person requests your help using an auto injector; and your state laws permit giving assistance.*

1. Check the label on the auto injector. If the medication is visible, check to make sure the medication is clear, not cloudy.

   ■ If the medication is expired or cloudy, do not use it.

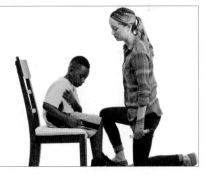

2. Determine whether the person has already given him- or herself a dose of the medication. If the person has, help him or her administer a second dose only if emergency responders are delayed and the person is still having signs and symptoms of anaphylaxis 5 to 10 minutes after administering the first dose.

3. Have the person locate the outer middle of one thigh to use as the injection site.

   ■ Make sure there is nothing in the way, such as seams or items in a pocket.

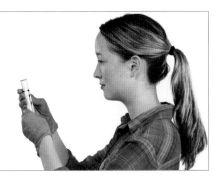

4. Grasp the auto injector firmly in one fist and pull off the safety cap with the other hand.

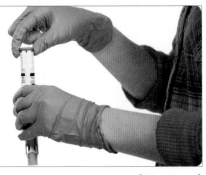

*(Continued)*

5.  Have the person hold the tip of the auto injector (the end with the needle) against his or her outer thigh so that the auto injector is at a 90-degree angle to the thigh.

6.  Have the person quickly and firmly push the tip straight into his or her outer thigh. You may hear a click. Have the person hold the auto injector firmly in place for the recommended amount of time.

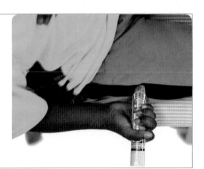

7.  Have the person remove the auto injector from his or her thigh. Massage the injection site for several seconds (or have the person massage the site).

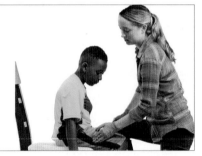

8.  Check the person's condition and watch to see how he or she responds to the medication.

    ■   If the person is still having signs and symptoms 5 to 10 minutes after administering the first dose and emergency responders have not arrived, help the person to administer a second dose.

9.  Place the used auto injector in its plastic carrying case or another hard plastic container with the tip facing down. Give it to the emergency responders when they arrive.

# 6

# TRAUMATIC INJURIES

The risk for injury is always present as we go about our daily activities and interact with the world around us. Taking appropriate safety precautions significantly reduces that risk, but injuries do happen. When a person is injured, providing proper first aid can speed recovery and may even save the person's life.

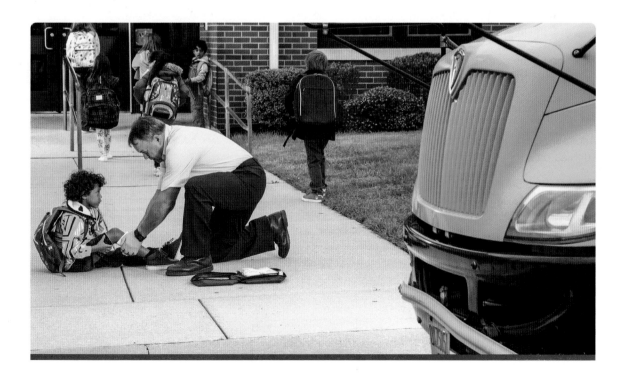

# Shock

**Shock** is a progressive, life-threatening condition in which the circulatory system fails to deliver enough oxygen-rich blood to the body's tissues and organs. As a result, organs and body systems begin to fail. Common causes of shock include severe bleeding and severe allergic reactions (anaphylaxis), but shock can develop quickly after any serious injury or illness. A person who is showing signs and symptoms of shock needs immediate medical attention.

## Signs and Symptoms of Shock

A person who is going into shock may show any of the following signs and symptoms:

- Restlessness or irritability

- Altered level of consciousness

- Nausea or vomiting

- Pale, ashen (grayish), cool, moist skin

- Rapid breathing

- Rapid, weak heartbeat

- Excessive thirst

## First Aid Care for Shock

When a person who has been injured or is ill shows signs and symptoms of shock, call 9-1-1 or the designated emergency number immediately, if you have not already done so. Shock cannot be managed effectively by first aid alone, so it is important to get the person emergency medical care as soon as possible. While you are waiting for help to arrive:

- Have the person lie flat on his or her back.

- Control any external bleeding.

- Cover the person with a blanket to prevent loss of body heat.

- Do not give the person anything to eat or drink, even though he or she may complain of thirst. Eating or drinking increases the person's risk for vomiting and aspiration (inhalation of foreign matter into the lungs). Aspiration can cause serious complications, such as pneumonia.

- Provide reassurance, and help the person rest comfortably. Anxiety and pain can intensify the body's stress and speed up the progression of shock.

- Continue to monitor the person's condition and watch for changes in level of consciousness.

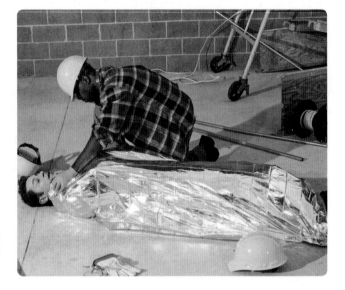

# Internal Bleeding

**Internal bleeding** (bleeding that occurs inside the body, into a body cavity or space) can be a consequence of traumatic injury and may be life threatening. **Blunt trauma**, which is caused by impact with a flat object or surface, is a common cause of internal bleeding. Mechanisms of injury that can lead to blunt trauma and internal bleeding include falls, being struck by a vehicle or a piece of heavy equipment, being struck by a blunt object (such as a bat) or being thrown into a blunt object (such as a steering wheel). Crushing forces (for example, when a person's body is squeezed between two hard surfaces) can also cause blunt trauma, leading to internal bleeding. **Penetrating trauma**, which occurs when the body is pierced by a sharp, narrow object (such as a knife or bullet) or impaled on a sharp object (such as a branch or piece of metal), can also lead to internal bleeding.

Internal bleeding may not be immediately obvious because the blood is contained within the body (e.g., within the abdomen, chest or skull). Often, when a person has sustained an injury that could cause internal bleeding, he or she will have other, more obvious injuries as well. When this is the case, medical treatment is usually sought for the more obvious injuries, and the internal bleeding is discovered while the person is being assessed by medical personnel. However, internal bleeding can also occur as a result of seemingly minor trauma, and it may reveal itself hours or days after the initial injury. When the mechanism of injury is one that could lead to internal bleeding (such as blunt or penetrating trauma), be alert to signs and symptoms that may indicate internal bleeding.

## Signs and Symptoms of Internal Bleeding

As a result of the blood loss, the person may show signs and symptoms of shock, such as excessive thirst; skin that feels cool or moist and looks pale or bluish; an altered level of consciousness; and a rapid, weak heartbeat. The person may cough or vomit blood. You may also notice that the area of the body where the blood is collecting (such as the abdomen) is tender, swollen or rigid, and there may be bruising over the area. If internal bleeding is occurring in an injured limb, the limb may be blue or extremely pale, swollen and rigid.

## First Aid Care for Internal Bleeding

If a person is showing signs and symptoms of internal bleeding, call 9-1-1 or the designated emergency number immediately, if you have not already done so. If necessary, give first aid care for shock until help arrives.

# Wounds

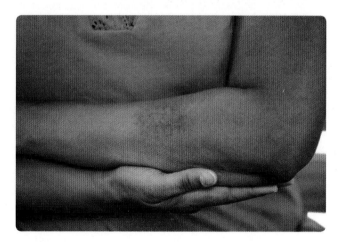

A **wound** is an injury that results when the skin or other tissues of the body are damaged. Wounds are generally classified as closed or open.

## Closed Wounds

When a person has a **closed wound**, the surface of the skin is intact but the underlying tissues are injured. A **bruise (contusion)** is a very common type of closed wound, usually caused by blunt trauma. Bruises occur when the small blood vessels under the surface of the skin are damaged and blood leaks into the surrounding tissues.

## Signs and Symptoms of Closed Wounds

The area may appear red or purple, and there may be swelling. The bruised area is often painful.

## First Aid Care for Closed Wounds

Applying a cold pack to the bruised area can help to decrease the bleeding and reduce pain and swelling. To make a cold pack, fill a sealable plastic bag with a mixture of ice and water. Before applying the cold pack to the person's skin, wrap it in a thin, dry towel to protect the skin from injury. Hold the cold pack in place for no more than 20 minutes, and then wait at least 20 minutes before applying the cold pack again. If the person is not able to tolerate a 20-minute application, apply the cold pack for periods of 10 minutes on and off. Elevating the injured area may help to reduce swelling, but do not elevate the injured area if doing so causes pain.

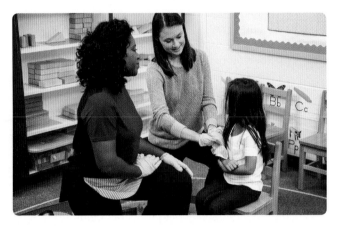

# Open Wounds

In an **open wound**, the skin's surface is broken and blood may come through the tear in the skin, resulting in **external bleeding** (bleeding that is visible on the outside of the body).

## Types of Open Wounds

The four main types of open wounds are abrasions, lacerations, avulsions and puncture wounds (Figure 6-1).

- An **abrasion** occurs when something rubs roughly against the skin, causing damage to the skin's surface. You may hear abrasions referred to as "scrapes," "rug burns," "road rash," or "turf burns." If you have ever had an abrasion, you know how painful these injuries can be! This is because scraping of the outer skin layers exposes sensitive nerve endings. Abrasions are shallow wounds that do not bleed much. However, because of the mechanism of injury (usually a sliding fall), abrasions are often contaminated with dirt and debris. To remove the dirt and debris, rinse the abrasion thoroughly with running water, and then wash the area with soap and water to lower the risk for infection.

- A **laceration** is a cut, commonly caused by a sharp object such as broken glass or a knife. A laceration can also occur when blunt force splits the skin. Deep lacerations may extend through layers of fat and muscle, damaging nerves, blood vessels and tendons. If nerves are damaged, the laceration may not be painful. Bleeding may be heavy or there may be none at all.

- An **avulsion** occurs when a portion of the skin, and sometimes the underlying tissue, is partially or completely torn away. Avulsions are commonly caused by animal bites. Elderly people are also susceptible to avulsion wounds as a result of a fall or other trauma because their skin is fragile and tears easily. Avulsion wounds often cause significant bleeding.

- A **puncture wound** occurs when a pointed object, such as a nail or an animal's tooth, pierces the skin. A gunshot wound is also a puncture wound. Puncture wounds do not bleed much unless a blood vessel has been injured. They carry a high risk for infection because the penetrating object can carry pathogens deep into the body's tissues.

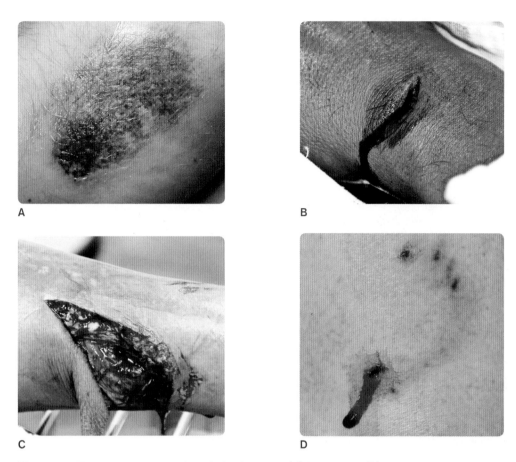

A

B

C

D

**Figure 6-1.** Types of open wounds include abrasions (A), lacerations (B), avulsions (C) and puncture wounds (D).

## First Aid Care for Open Wounds

Many open wounds are minor and can be cared for effectively using first aid. However, if the wound is deep or extensive, bleeding heavily or uncontrollably, or carries a high risk for infection (e.g., a puncture wound), medical care will be needed (Box 6-1).

## Minor Open Wounds

To care for a minor open wound, put on latex-free disposable gloves and other personal protective equipment (PPE) as necessary. Apply direct pressure with a gauze pad to stop the bleeding. It may take several minutes for the bleeding to stop. After the bleeding stops, wash the area with soap and warm water. Rinse under warm running water for about 5 minutes until the wound appears clean and free of debris, and then dry the area. Apply a small amount of antibiotic ointment, cream or gel to the wound if the person has no known allergies or sensitivities to the ingredients. Then cover the area with a sterile gauze pad and a bandage, or apply an adhesive bandage. When you are finished providing care, wash your hands with soap and water, even if you wore gloves.

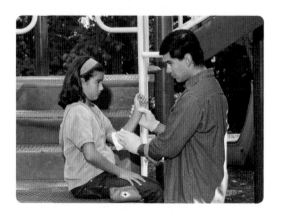

**Myth-Information.** *Myth: Use hydrogen peroxide to clean a wound and prevent infection; the bubbles mean it is working to kill germs.* Although applying hydrogen peroxide to a wound will kill germs, it also can harm the tissue and delay healing. The best way to clean a wound is with soap and warm, running water or saline.

# Box 6-1. **Does This Wound Need Medical Attention?**

Depending on the cause of the wound and the nature of the injury, it may be necessary to see a healthcare provider for treatment.

## Tetanus Prophylaxis

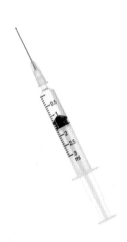

When a wound is deep or dirty, you should seek care from a healthcare provider, especially if you do not know or cannot remember when you last had a tetanus booster shot, or if it has been more than 5 years since your last tetanus booster shot. **Tetanus** is a severe bacterial infection that can result from a puncture wound or a deep laceration. The bacteria that cause tetanus are commonly found in soil and animal manure. Once introduced into the body via a deep or dirty wound, they produce a powerful toxin that can cause muscle paralysis and death. Signs and symptoms of tetanus infection include muscle spasms and stiffness. The spasms and stiffness begin in the jaw and neck, leading to difficulty swallowing (a classic sign of tetanus). As the infection progresses, the muscle spasms and weakness spread to the abdomen and then to the rest of the body.

Although the effects of the tetanus toxin can be managed through administration of an antitoxin, prevention through immunization is a better strategy. The initial tetanus vaccine series is usually given during childhood, and then immunity is maintained through a booster shot given at least every 10 years. Death rates from tetanus infection are highest among those who were never immunized against tetanus and those who fail to maintain adequate immunization through regular booster shots.

## Placement of Stitches

Suturing a wound closed can speed the healing process, reduce the chance for infection and minimize scarring. Stitches should be placed within the first few hours after the injury. If you think that a wound needs stitches, it probably does. If in doubt, have the wound evaluated by a healthcare provider. In general, the following types of wounds often require stitches:

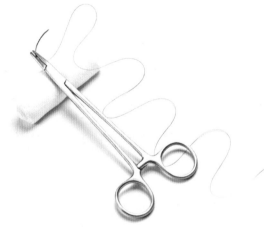

- Wounds that are deep or longer than ½ inch

- Wounds on parts of the body where scarring could impair appearance or function (for example, the face, hands or feet)

- Wounds caused by human or animal bites

- Wounds with jagged edges that gape open

- Wounds that are bleeding heavily and uncontrollably

*(Continued)*

# Treatment of Infection

Proper wound care helps to lower the risk for infection, but sometimes infections develop anyway. An untreated wound infection can cause complications, including delayed wound healing; infection of nearby skin (cellulitis) or bone (osteomyelitis); or infection throughout the body (sepsis, which can be fatal). See your healthcare provider if you notice signs and symptoms of infection or if the wound does not seem to be healing. Signs and symptoms of an infected wound may include:

■ Increased pain, swelling, redness or warmth in the area of the wound.

■ Red streaks extending from the area of the wound.

■ Pus (a thick yellow or green fluid) draining from the wound.

■ Fever.

The healthcare provider may use advanced wound-care strategies, antibiotics or both to eliminate the infection and promote wound healing.

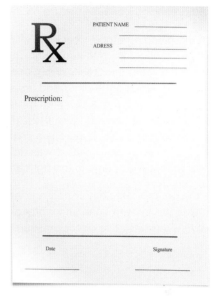

**Myth-Information.** *Myth: Letting a wound "breathe" by exposing it to air helps it to heal.* A better strategy to promote wound healing is to keep the wound moist (with an antibiotic ointment, cream or gel) and covered (under a dressing and bandage).

## Major Open Wounds

A major open wound (for example, one that involves extensive tissue damage or is bleeding heavily or uncontrollably) requires prompt action. Call 9-1-1 or the designated emergency number immediately and then take steps to control the bleeding until help arrives.

### Applying Direct Pressure

Put on latex-free disposable gloves and other personal protective equipment (PPE) as necessary (for example, if blood is spurting, you may need to wear eye and face protection). Cover the area with a

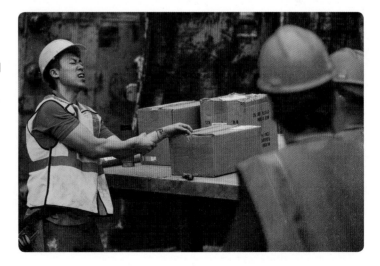

sterile gauze pad or other clean dressing (Box 6-2) and apply direct pressure with your gloved hand until the bleeding stops. This may take as long as 15 minutes. If blood soaks through the first dressing, place another dressing on top of the first and apply additional direct pressure (press harder than you did before, if possible). Repeat with additional dressings as needed, always maintaining direct pressure. Do not remove the blood-soaked dressings because disturbing them may disrupt clot formation and restart the bleeding.

When the bleeding stops, check the skin on the side of the injury farthest away from the heart (e.g., the hand or foot) for feeling, warmth and color. Then apply a bandage over the dressing to maintain pressure on the wound and to hold the dressing in place. To apply a roller bandage, hold one end of the roller bandage in place while you wrap the other end around the wound and dressing several times, using overlapping turns. Make sure the dressing is completely covered and allow a margin of several inches on all sides. Tie or tape the bandage to secure it (Figure 6-2). The bandage should be snug but not too tight. Check for feeling, warmth and color again. If there is a change in feeling, warmth or color from your first check (for example, the skin is cooler or paler than it was before, the area is swollen, or the person complains of a numb or tingly feeling), then the bandage is too tight and needs to be loosened.

Have the person rest comfortably and provide care for shock, if necessary, until help arrives. Remember to wash your hands with soap and water after providing care, even if you wore gloves. Skill Sheet 6-1 describes step by step how to use direct pressure to control external bleeding.

## Box 6-2. **Dressings and Bandages**

Dressings and bandages are staples of any well-stocked first aid kit and have a variety of uses.

### Dressings

A **dressing** is a pad that is placed directly on a wound to absorb blood and other fluids, promote clotting and prevent infection. To minimize the chance of infection, dressings should be sterile. There are many different types of dressings available. In a first aid situation, gauze pads, which are available in a variety of sizes, are most commonly used as dressings.

### Bandages

A **bandage** is a strip of material used to hold the dressing in place and to control bleeding. Roller bandages, made of gauze or a gauze-like material, are frequently included in first aid kits and come in a variety of widths and lengths. Wrap the bandage around the injured body part, covering the dressing completely and allowing a margin of several inches on all sides. Then tie or tape the bandage to secure it in place. Bandage compresses, which are specially designed to control severe bleeding and usually come in sterile packages, are thick gauze dressings attached to a bandage that is tied in place.

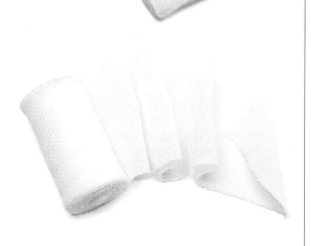

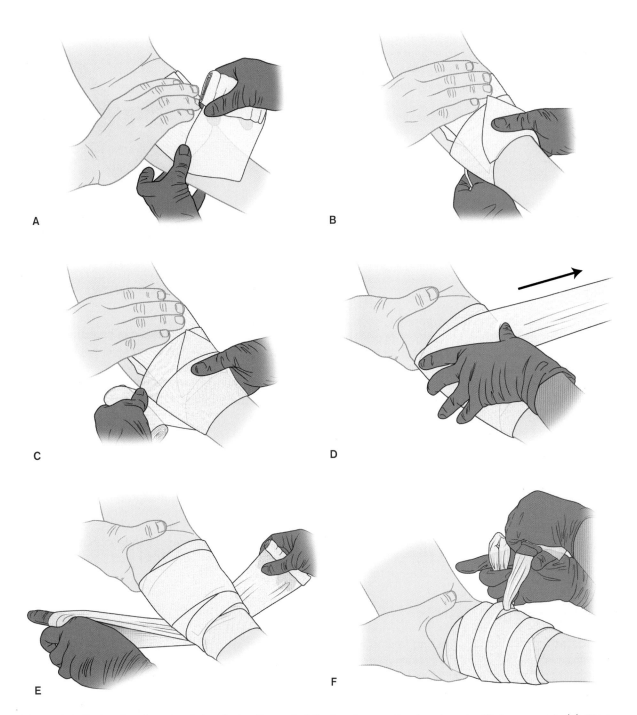

**Figure 6-2.** To tie a bandage, begin by placing the end of the bandage on the dressing at a 45-degree angle (A). Wrap the bandage one full turn, and then fold the angled end of the bandage up, creating a "dog ear" (B). Continue wrapping the bandage, overlaying the "dog ear" to anchor it and moving upward (C). Once the dressing is covered, roll out the remaining length of bandage (D). While holding the bandage, use the index finger of the other hand to split the bandage in half, moving it down and underneath the limb (E). Bring the two ends of the bandage up and tie them in a bow or knot (F).

## Applying a Tourniquet

A **tourniquet** is a device placed around an arm or leg to constrict blood vessels and stop blood flow to a wound. In some life-threatening circumstances, you may need to use a tourniquet to control bleeding as the first step instead of maintaining direct pressure over several minutes. Examples of situations where it may be necessary to use a tourniquet include:

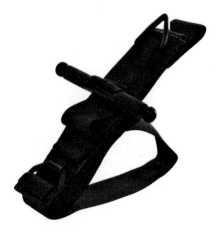

- Severe, life-threatening bleeding that cannot be controlled using direct pressure.

- A physical location that makes it impossible to apply direct pressure to control the bleeding (e.g., the injured person or the person's limb is trapped in a confined space).

- Multiple people with life-threatening injuries who need care.

- A scene that is or becomes unsafe.

**THE PROS KNOW.**

———

Tourniquets can be extremely painful. If you must apply a tourniquet, make sure the person understands the reason for the tourniquet, and warn the person that it may be painful.

If you find yourself in a situation where you need to apply a tourniquet, a commercially manufactured tourniquet is preferred over a makeshift device. Follow the manufacturer's instructions for applying the tourniquet. Although tourniquets may have slightly different designs, all are applied in generally the same way. First, place the tourniquet around the wounded extremity about 2 inches above the wound, avoiding the joint if possible. Secure the tourniquet tightly in place according to the manufacturer's instructions. Twist the rod (windlass) to tighten the tourniquet until the bright red bleeding stops, then secure the rod in place. Note and record the time that you applied the tourniquet and be sure to give EMS personnel this information when they arrive. Once the tourniquet is applied, it should not be removed until the person reaches a healthcare facility. Skill Sheet 6-2 describes step by step how to apply a commercially manufactured tourniquet.

If it is necessary to use a tourniquet and a commercially manufactured tourniquet is not available, make a tourniquet using a strip of soft material that is 2 to 4 inches wide (such as a triangular bandage that has been folded into a tie) and a short, sturdy stick or other rigid object. Tie the stick or other rigid object into the material and twist it to tighten the makeshift tourniquet.

## Using Hemostatic Dressings

A **hemostatic dressing** is a dressing treated with a substance that speeds clot formation. As is the case with tourniquets, hemostatic dressings are used when severe life-threatening bleeding exists and standard first aid procedures fail or are not practical. Typically, hemostatic dressings are used on parts of the body where a tourniquet cannot be applied, such as the neck or torso. A hemostatic dressing can also be used to control bleeding from an open wound on an arm or a leg if a tourniquet is ineffective. The hemostatic dressing is applied at the site of the bleeding (possibly inside of the wound) and is used along with direct pressure.

## Open Wounds with Embedded Objects

In some cases, the object that caused the wound may remain in the wound. If the embedded object is large (for example, a large piece of glass or metal), do not attempt to remove it. Instead, place several dressings around the object to begin to control blood loss, and then pack bulk dressings or roller bandages around the embedded object to keep it from moving. Bandage the bulk dressings or roller bandages in place around the object and seek medical care. Remember to monitor the person for signs and symptoms of shock.

A small partially embedded object, such as a splinter, can usually be removed using first aid techniques; however, medical care should be sought if the splinter is deep, completely embedded in the skin, or located under the nail or in the eye. To remove a simple shallow splinter, grasp the end of the splinter with clean tweezers and pull it out. Then provide care as you would for any minor open wound.

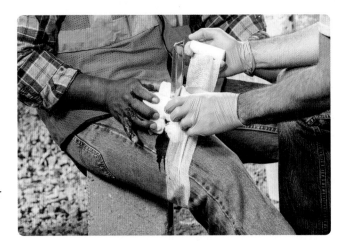

## Traumatic Amputations

Traumatic amputation is the loss of a body part as a result of an injury. Common causes of traumatic amputations include injuries involving power tools, farming or manufacturing equipment; motor-vehicle collisions; explosions and natural disasters. In a traumatic amputation, the body part might be severed cleanly from the body or ripped away as a result of being subjected to violent tearing or twisting forces. Crushing forces can also result in mangled tissue and traumatic amputations. The body part may be completely detached from the body, or it may still be partially attached. Bleeding may be minimal or severe, depending on the location and nature of the injury.

When a person has experienced a traumatic amputation, call 9-1-1 or the designated emergency number. If the body part is completely detached from the body, try to locate it because surgeons may be able to reattach it. Wrap the amputated body part in sterile gauze or other clean material. Put the wrapped body part in a plastic bag and seal the bag. Keep the bag containing the body part cool by placing it in a larger bag or container filled with a mixture of ice and water. Do not place the bag containing the body part directly on ice or dry ice. Give the bag containing the body part to EMS personnel so that it can be taken to the hospital along with the person.

# Burns

A **burn** is a traumatic injury to the skin (and sometimes the underlying tissues as well) caused by contact with extreme heat, chemicals, radiation or electricity (Figure 6-3).

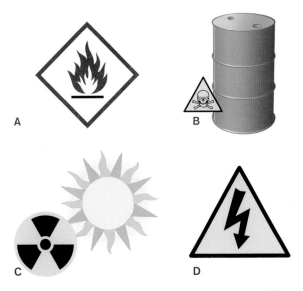

**Figure 6-3. Causes of burns include extreme heat (A), chemicals (B), radiation (C) and electricity (D).**

Burns range in severity from minor to critical. A critical burn is one that is life threatening or potentially disfiguring or disabling, and it requires immediate medical attention. When evaluating whether a burn is critical or not, consider the following factors:

- **The depth of the burn.** Burns can be classified according to depth (Figure 6-4). Superficial burns only involve the epidermis (the top layer of skin). Partial-thickness burns involve the epidermis and the dermis (the layer of skin underneath the epidermis that contains blood vessels, nerves, hair follicles and glands). Full-thickness burns involve both layers of skin and may extend into the subcutaneous tissue, muscle or bone underneath. Generally speaking, the deeper the burn, the greater the severity.

- **The percentage of the body's surface area that is burned.** A burn that covers more than one part of the body or covers a large percentage of the person's total body surface area requires medical attention. Even a superficial burn can be a critical burn if it affects a large percentage of the person's total body surface area.

- **The location of the burn.** Burns that affect the hands, feet or groin; those that involve the head, neck, nose, or mouth or affect the person's ability to breathe; and circumferential burns (i.e., those that go all the way around a limb) are considered critical burns.

- **The age of the person.** If the person is younger than 5 years or older than 60 years, the burn should be considered critical, unless it is very minor.

- **The cause of the burn.** Burns caused by electricity, exposure to chemicals, exposure to nuclear radiation or an explosion are considered critical burns.

If you think that a person has a critical burn, call 9-1-1 or the designated emergency number immediately.

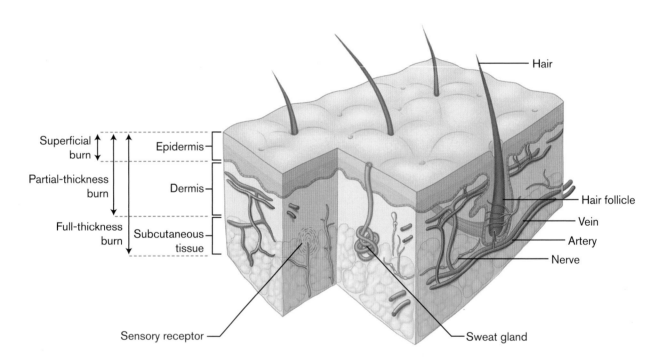

**Figure 6-4. Burns can be classified according to depth.**

# Signs and Symptoms of Burns

Burned areas can appear red, brown, black (charred) or white. The burned area may be extremely painful or almost painless (if the burn is deep enough to destroy the nerve endings). There may be swelling, blisters or both. The blisters may break and ooze a clear fluid. Burns involving blistering or broken skin should be evaluated by a healthcare provider.

# First Aid Care for Burns

**Myth-Information.** *Myth: Soothe a burn with butter.* Not a good idea! Putting butter, mayonnaise, petroleum jelly or any other greasy substance on a burn is not effective for relieving pain or promoting healing. In fact, applying a greasy substance to the burn can seal in the heat and make the burn worse.

First aid for burns involves three general steps—stop, cool and cover:

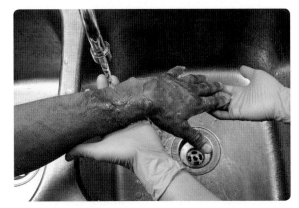

- **Stop.** First, after sizing up the scene, stop the burning by removing the source of the injury if it is safe for you to do so. Depending on the cause of the burn, this may involve removing the person from the source or removing the source from the person.

- **Cool.** Next, cool the burn and relieve pain using clean, cool or cold water for at least 10 minutes. Use water that you could drink. Never use ice or ice water to cool a burn because doing so can cause more damage to the skin. If clean cool or cold water is not available, you can apply a cool or cold (but not freezing) compress instead. Cooling a burn over a large area of the body can bring on hypothermia (a body temperature below normal), so be alert to signs and symptoms of this condition (see Chapter 7).

- **Cover.** Finally, cover the burn loosely with a sterile dressing. Make sure that whatever you use to cover the wound is sterile or at least clean, because burns leave the person highly susceptible to infection.

Burns of all types, especially if they cover a large percentage of the body, can cause a person to go into shock, so monitor the person closely. When caring for a burn, do not remove pieces of clothing that are stuck to the burned area, do not attempt to clean a severe burn and do not break any blisters.

## Chemical Burns

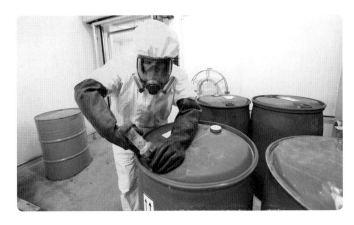

The general care for a chemical burn is the same as for any other type of burn: stop, cool, cover. However, there are some special considerations for the "stop" step. Because the chemical will continue to burn as long as it is on the skin, you must remove the chemical from the skin as quickly as possible.

- **Dry chemicals.** If the burn was caused by a dry chemical, such as lime, brush off the powder or granules with gloved hands or a cloth, being careful not to get any of the chemical on your skin or on a different area of the person's skin. Carefully remove, or help the person to remove, any clothing that was contaminated with the chemical. Then flush the area thoroughly with large amounts of cool water for at least 15 minutes or until EMS personnel arrive.

- **Liquid chemicals.** If the burn resulted from a liquid chemical coming into contact with the skin, flush the affected area with large amounts of cool water for at least 15 minutes or until EMS personnel arrive.

If the chemical is in the person's eye, flush the eye with water until EMS personnel arrive. Tilt the person's head so that the affected eye is lower than the unaffected eye as you flush.

## Electrical Burns

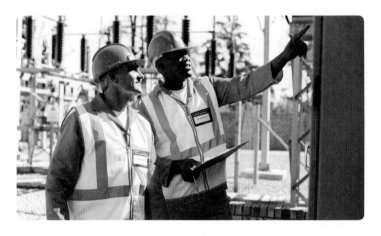

First aid for electrical burns also follows the general principle of "stop, cool, cover," but as with chemical burns, there are some special care considerations when electricity is the cause of the burn. As always, check the scene for safety before entering. Make sure 9-1-1 or the designated emergency number has been called, and if possible, turn off the power at its source. Do not approach or touch the person until you are sure he or she is no longer in contact with the electrical current. Once you have determined that it is safe to approach the person, provide care as needed until help arrives. Because the electrical current that caused the burns can also affect the heart's rhythm or the person's ability to breathe (causing the person to go into cardiac arrest), be prepared to give CPR and use an AED if you are trained in these skills.

Anyone who has experienced an electrical burn should be evaluated by a healthcare provider because the person's injuries may be more extensive than they appear. Although the person may only have a small burn wound where the electrical current entered or left the body, there may be significant internal injuries caused by the current passing through the body.

# Muscle, Bone and Joint Injuries

Injuries to the muscles, bones and joints include sprains, strains, dislocations and fractures.

- A **sprain** occurs when a ligament is stretched, torn or damaged. Ligaments connect bones to bones at the joints. Sprains most commonly affect the ankle, knee, wrist and finger joints.

- A **strain** occurs when a tendon or muscle is stretched, torn or damaged. Tendons connect muscles to bones. Strains often are caused by lifting something heavy or working a muscle too hard. They usually involve the muscles in the neck, back, thigh or the back of the lower leg. Some strains can reoccur, especially in the neck and back.

- A **dislocation** occurs when the bones that meet at a joint move out of their normal position. This type of injury is usually caused by a violent force that tears the ligaments, allowing the bones to move out of place.

- A **fracture** is a complete break, a chip or a crack in a bone. Fractures can be open (the end of the broken bone breaks through the skin) or closed (the broken bone does not break through the skin).

# Signs and Symptoms of Muscle, Bone and Joint Injuries

Muscle, bone and joint injuries can be extremely painful. Sometimes the injury will be very obvious—for example, you may see the ends of a broken bone protruding through the skin, or the injured body part might appear bent or crooked (deformed). If a joint is dislocated, you may see an abnormal bump, ridge or hollow formed by the displaced end of the bone. Other times, signs and symptoms of injury may be more subtle, such as swelling or bruising. Usually, the person will try to avoid using the injured body part because using it causes pain. In some cases, the person may be unable to move the injured body part. The person might also report feeling or hearing "popping" or "snapping" at the time of the injury, or "grating" when moving the injured part.

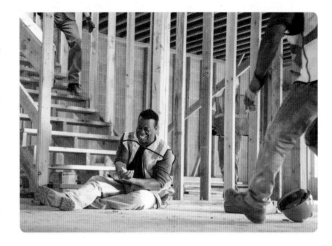

Sometimes when a person has a muscle, bone or joint injury, you will be able to tell right away that you need to call 9-1-1 or the designated emergency number. But not all muscle, bone or joint injuries result in obvious injuries, and some are not serious enough to summon emergency medical services (EMS) personnel. In general, call 9-1-1 or the designated emergency number if:

- A broken bone is protruding through the skin.

- The injured body part is bent, crooked or looks deformed.

- There is moderate or severe swelling and bruising.

- The person heard or felt "popping" or "snapping" at the time of the injury.

- The person hears or feels "grating" when he or she moves the injured body part.

- The person cannot move or use the injured body part.

- The injured area is cold and numb.

- The injury involves the head, neck or spine.

- The person is having difficulty breathing.

- The cause of the injury (for example, a fall from a height or getting hit by a vehicle) makes you think that the injury may be severe, or that the person may have multiple injuries.

- It is not possible to safely or comfortably move the person to a vehicle for transport to a healthcare facility.

# First Aid Care for Muscle, Bone and Joint Injuries

If you have called 9-1-1 or the designated emergency number and are waiting for EMS personnel to arrive, have the person rest without moving or straightening the body part. If the person can tolerate it, apply a cold pack wrapped in a thin, dry towel to the area to reduce swelling and pain.

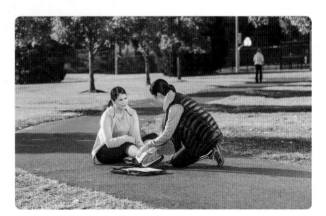

## RICE

In some cases, it may only be necessary for the person to see his or her healthcare provider to have the injury evaluated. If calling EMS is unnecessary, the mnemonic RICE can help you remember how to care for a muscle, bone or joint injury:

- **R** stands for *rest.* Limit use of the injured body part.

- **I** stands for *immobilize.* Stabilize the injured body part with an elastic bandage or a splint to limit motion.

- **C** stands for *cold.* Apply a cold pack wrapped in a thin, dry towel to the area for no more than 20 minutes at a time, and wait at least 20 minutes before applying the cold pack again.

- **E** stands for *elevate.* Propping the injured part up may help to reduce swelling, but do not do this if raising the injured part causes more pain.

**Myth-Information.** *Myth: Apply heat to a muscle, bone or joint injury to speed healing.* Although applying heat is commonly used to relieve pain associated with chronic muscle, bone and joint conditions such as arthritis, it is not the best treatment for an acute muscle, bone or joint injury. Applying heat causes the blood vessels in the area to dilate (widen), bringing more blood to the area and increasing swelling. Cold, on the other hand, causes blood vessels to constrict (narrow), reducing blood flow to the area, helping to reduce swelling. In addition, applying cold slows nerve impulses, helping to reduce pain.

## Splinting

Splinting is a way to prevent movement of an injured bone or joint. It can also help reduce pain. However, you should only apply a splint if you *must* move the person to get medical help, and if splinting does not cause the person more pain or discomfort.

Splinting involves securing the injured body part to the splint to keep it from moving. Commercial splints are available. You can also make a splint using soft materials (such as blankets, towels or pillows) or rigid materials (such as a folded magazine or a board). You can even use an adjacent part of the body as a splint (for example, you can splint an injured finger to the uninjured finger next to it). This is called an anatomic splint.

Triangular bandages are handy to keep in your first aid kit in case you need to make a splint. A triangular bandage can be used to make a sling (a special kind of splint that is used to hold an injured arm against the chest) and to make ties to hold other kinds of splints in place. A "cravat fold" is used to turn a triangular bandage into a tie (Figure 6-5).

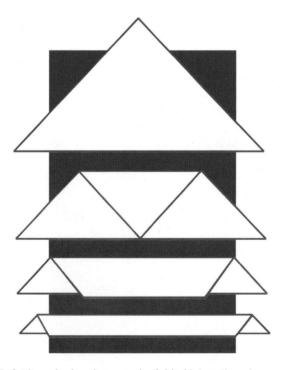

**Figure 6-5. A triangular bandage can be folded into a tie using a cravat fold.**

The general rules for applying a splint are the same no matter what type of splint you use:

- Splint the body part in the position in which you found it. Do not try to straighten or move the body part.

- Make sure the splint is long enough to extend above and below the injured area. If a joint is injured, include the bones above and below the joint in the splint. If a bone is injured, include the joints above and below the bone in the splint. If you are not sure what is injured, include both the bones and the joints above and below the injured area in the splint.

- Check for feeling, warmth and color beyond the site of injury before and after splinting to make sure that the splint is not too tight.

# Head, Neck and Spinal Injuries

Traumatic accidents (such as falling from a height, getting hit by or being thrown from a vehicle, or sustaining a blow to the head) can cause head, neck or spinal injuries. Head, neck or spinal injuries are serious because they may involve the spinal cord or the brain. Depending on the nature and severity of the injury, the person may be left with a permanent disability (e.g., traumatic brain injury, paralysis). Some head, neck or spinal injuries are fatal.

- **Spinal cord injuries** can result from trauma that causes one or more vertebrae (the bones that surround and protect the spinal cord) to break. The sharp bone fragments can press into the soft tissue of the spinal cord, damaging it. Damage can also occur if the injury causes the soft tissue of the spinal cord to swell, compressing it against the hard bone that surrounds it. Depending on the location and severity of the spinal cord injury, the person may develop **paralysis** (the loss of movement, sensation or both) in body parts below the level of the injury. **Paraplegia** is paralysis that affects both legs and the lower trunk. **Quadriplegia** is paralysis that affects both arms, the trunk and both legs.

- **Brain injuries** can occur as a result of a blow to the head, a penetrating injury to the head (such as a bullet wound), or exposure to acceleration-deceleration forces that cause the head to snap forward and then back. A blow to the head can lead to a **concussion** (a traumatic brain injury that alters the way the brain functions; Box 6-3), a **brain contusion** (bruising of the brain tissue) or a **brain hematoma** (bleeding into the space between the brain and the skull). Acceleration-deceleration forces, such as can occur with a motor-vehicle collision or a fall from a height, can lead to **diffuse axonal injury** (tearing of nerves throughout the brain tissue).

## Causes of Head, Neck and Spinal Injuries

Many different types of accidents can lead to head, neck or spinal injuries. You should especially consider the possibility of a head, neck or spinal injury if the person:

- Was hit by a vehicle, thrown from a moving vehicle, or was the occupant of a vehicle involved in a motor-vehicle collision.

- Was injured as a result of entering shallow water headfirst.

- Was injured as a result of a fall from a height greater than his or her own height.

- Was participating in a sport and sustained a blow to the head or collided with another player, the ground or a piece of equipment.

# Box 6-3. **Concussions**

A concussion is a common type of traumatic brain injury that involves a temporary loss of brain function. Concussions are particularly common sports-related injuries, but they can occur whenever a person experiences a bump, blow or jolt to the head or body that results in rapid movement of the head. A person who has had one concussion is at increased risk for subsequent concussions.

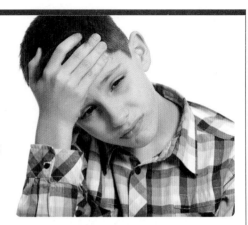

A concussion can result from even a seemingly minor bump, blow or jolt and may be tricky to recognize. Many people who experience a concussion do not lose consciousness, or they may only lose consciousness very briefly. Your best clues that a person may have a concussion are often changes in the person's behavior noted after the person has experienced a bump, blow or jolt. For example, the person may seem confused, dazed or stunned; lose the ability to remember or follow simple instructions; or ask repeatedly what happened. The person may complain of a headache, feel nauseated or vomit, have blurred or double vision, complain of dizziness, or be especially sensitive to light or noise. Many people who have experienced a concussion say that the concussion caused them to feel "sluggish," "groggy" or just "not right." Signs and symptoms of a concussion usually are apparent soon after the injury, although some can appear hours or days later. For example, the person may sleep more or less than usual. Children may show changes in playing or eating habits. The effects of the concussion can last for several days, weeks or longer.

## Signs and Symptoms of Concussion

| Thinking and Remembering | Physical | Emotional | Behavioral |
|---|---|---|---|
| ■ Difficulty thinking clearly<br>■ Difficulty remembering events that occurred just prior to the incident and just after the incident<br>■ Difficulty remembering new information<br>■ Difficulty concentrating<br>■ Feeling mentally "foggy"<br>■ Difficulty processing information | ■ Headache<br>■ Blurry vision<br>■ Nausea or vomiting<br>■ Dizziness<br>■ Sensitivity to noise or light<br>■ Balance problems<br>■ Feeling sluggish (lack of energy) | ■ Irritability<br>■ Sadness<br>■ Heightened emotions<br>■ Nervousness or anxiety | ■ Changes in sleeping habits (sleeping more or less than usual, difficulty falling asleep)<br>■ Changes in playing and eating habits (in children) |

If you think that a person has sustained a concussion, advise the person to stop the activity he or she was engaged in when the incident occurred. The person should follow up with a healthcare provider for a full evaluation. A healthcare provider is best able to evaluate the severity of the injury and make recommendations about when the person can return to normal activities. And, while rare, permanent brain injury and death are potential consequences of failing to identify and respond to a concussion in a timely manner.

> **Myth-Information.** *Myth: A person with a concussion who falls asleep could die.* It is generally considered safe for a person with a concussion to go to sleep. However, the person's healthcare provider may recommend that you wake the person periodically to make sure that his or her condition has not worsened.

# Signs and Symptoms of Head, Neck and Spinal Injuries

The signs and symptoms of a head, neck or spinal injury depend on the nature and location of the injury, but could include:

- Unusual bumps, bruises or depressions on the head, neck or back.

- Heavy external bleeding of the head, neck or back.

- Bruising of the head, especially around the eyes and behind the ears.

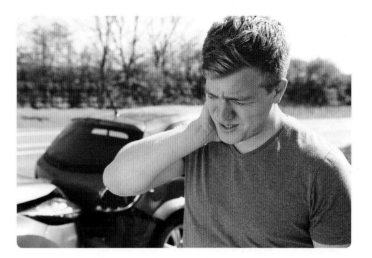

- Blood or other fluids in the ears or nose.

- Confusion or disorientation.

- Changes in level of consciousness.

- Seizures.

- Impaired breathing or vision.

- Nausea or vomiting.

- Partial or complete loss of movement of any body part.

- Loss of balance.

- Behavior similar to that of a person under the influence of alcohol or drugs (e.g., confusion, stumbling, repeatedly asking the same questions, memory loss, nausea or vomiting, speech problems).

- Severe pain or pressure in the head, neck or back (reported by the person or indicated by the person holding his or her head, neck or back).

- Back pain, weakness, tingling or loss of sensation in the hands, fingers, feet or toes.

- Persistent headache.

- A broken or damaged safety helmet.

# First Aid Care for Head, Neck and Spinal Injuries

Because evaluation by medical personnel is needed to determine the severity of a head, neck or spinal injury, you should always assume that an injury involving the head, neck or spine is serious and provide care accordingly. If you suspect a head, neck or spinal injury, call 9-1-1 or the designated emergency number. As long as the person is breathing normally, have him or her remain in the position in which he or she was found. If the person is wearing a helmet, do not remove it unless you are specifically trained to do so and removing the helmet is necessary to give CPR. Similarly, if a child is strapped into a car seat, do not remove him or her from it unless you need to give the child CPR.

**THE PROS KNOW.**

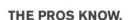

If you suspect that a person has a head, neck or spinal injury, approach the person from the front so that he or she can see you without turning his or her head. Tell the person to respond verbally to your questions, rather than nodding or shaking his or her head.

# Nose and Mouth Injuries

Facial trauma can range from minor injuries (cuts and abrasions, bruises, bloody noses and knocked-out teeth) to more severe injuries, such as a fracture of one or more of the facial bones. A person with a facial injury may also have a head, neck or spinal injury, such as a concussion.

## Nose Injuries

Falling or getting hit in the nose can result in a nosebleed. Other, nontraumatic causes of nosebleeds include breathing dry air and changes in altitude. Certain medical conditions (such as hypertension, or high blood pressure) and the use of certain medications (such as blood thinners) can make a person more susceptible to nosebleeds.

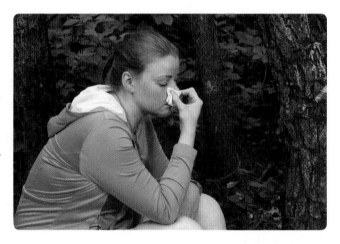

In most cases, you can stop a nosebleed by having the person pinch his or her nostrils together while sitting with his or her head slightly forward. (Sitting with the head slightly forward helps to keep blood from pooling in the back of the throat, which can lead to choking or, if the blood is swallowed, vomiting.) Keep the nostrils pinched shut for at least 5 minutes before checking to see if the bleeding has stopped. If the bleeding has not stopped after 5 minutes, keep pinching the nostrils shut for another 5 minutes. If the bleeding is severe or gushing, call 9-1-1 or the designated emergency number.

## Mouth Injuries

Injuries to the mouth may cause breathing problems if blood or loose teeth block the airway, so make sure the person is able to breathe. If the person is bleeding from the mouth and you do not suspect a serious head, neck or spinal injury, place the person in a seated position leaning slightly forward. This will allow any blood to drain from the mouth. If this position is not possible, place the person on his or her side in the recovery position. Have the person hold a gauze pad at the site of the bleeding and apply direct pressure to stop the bleeding. (If the person is responsive, having the person apply direct pressure to a wound inside his or her own mouth is easier and safer than doing it for the person.)

### Lip and Tongue Injuries

For injuries that penetrate the lip, place a rolled gauze pad between the lip and the gum. You can place another gauze pad on the outer surface of the lip. If the tongue is bleeding, apply a gauze pad and direct pressure. Applying a cold pack wrapped in a dry towel to the lips or tongue can help to reduce swelling and ease pain.

### Dental Injuries

If a tooth is knocked out, control the bleeding by placing a rolled gauze pad into the space left by the missing tooth and have the person gently bite down to maintain pressure. Try to locate and save the tooth, because a dentist or other healthcare provider may be able to reimplant it. Place the tooth in Hanks' Balanced Salt solution (e.g., Save-A-Tooth®), if available. If you do not have Hanks' Balanced Salt solution, place the tooth in egg white, coconut water or whole milk. If these are not available, place the tooth in the injured person's saliva. Be careful to pick up the tooth only by the crown (the part of the tooth that is normally visible above the gumline) rather than by the root. The person should seek dental or emergency care as soon as possible after the injury. The sooner the tooth is reimplanted, the better the chance that it will survive. Ideally, reimplantation should take place within 30 minutes.

# Chest Injuries

The chest cavity contains the heart, the major blood vessels that enter and leave the heart, the lungs, the trachea and most of the esophagus. These vital organs are protected by a bony cage formed by the ribs and breastbone (sternum). Chest injuries may involve the organs and major blood vessels housed in the chest cavity, the bones that form the chest cavity, or both.

Traumatic chest injuries are frequently caused by blunt trauma. Penetrating trauma (e.g., a stab or gunshot wound) is also a common cause of traumatic chest injuries. Internal bleeding is likely when a person has sustained significant trauma to the chest.

- **Rib fractures** are a common chest injury associated with blunt trauma. Although painful, a simple broken rib rarely is life threatening. Broken ribs are less common in children than in adults because children's ribs are more flexible and tend to bend rather than break. However, the forces that can cause a broken rib in adults can severely bruise the lung tissue of children, which can be a life-threatening injury.

- **Flail chest** occurs when multiple ribs are broken in more than one place, usually as a result of severe blunt trauma. This interferes with the mechanics of breathing because the injured area is not able to expand properly. (Expansion of the chest is what draws air into the lungs.) Flail chest is also frequently associated with a **lung contusion** (bruising of the lung tissue), which can be life threatening.

- **Sucking chest wounds** can occur as a result of penetrating trauma. The puncture wound can allow air to enter the space between the lung and the chest wall. The abnormal collection of air in this space puts pressure on the lung, causing it to collapse (a condition called **pneumothorax**). In addition to putting the person at risk for pneumothorax, the object that caused the puncture wound can injure the organs or vessels contained within the chest cavity and cause varying degrees of internal or external bleeding.

## Signs and Symptoms of Chest Injuries

A person with a broken rib may take small, shallow breaths because normal or deep breathing is uncomfortable or painful. The person usually will attempt to ease the pain by supporting the injured area with a hand or arm.

Signs and symptoms of a more serious chest injury (such as multiple broken ribs, internal bleeding, a lung contusion or a sucking chest wound) could include:

- Difficulty breathing.

- Flushed, pale, ashen or bluish skin.

- Severe pain at the site of the injury.

- Bruising at the site of a blunt injury, such as that caused by a seat belt.

- Deformity of the chest wall.

- Unusual movement of the chest wall when the person breathes, which may include **paradoxical breathing** (when the person inhales, the injured area draws in while the rest of the chest expands, and when the person exhales, the injured area expands while the rest of the chest draws in) or movement of only one side of the chest.

- Coughing up blood, which may be bright red or dark like coffee grounds.

- A "sucking" sound coming from the wound with each breath the person takes (caused by air entering the chest cavity through an open chest wound).

- Signs and symptoms of shock, such as excessive thirst; skin that feels cool or moist and looks pale or bluish; an altered level of consciousness; and a rapid, weak heartbeat.

If the person is showing signs and symptoms of a serious chest injury, or you think that the person might also have a spinal injury, call 9-1-1 or the designated emergency number.

# First Aid Care for Chest Injuries

First aid care for a chest injury depends on the type of injury.

## Rib Fracture

Give the person a pillow or folded blanket to hold against the injured area to provide support and make breathing more comfortable. The person should be evaluated by a healthcare provider, so call 9-1-1 or the designated emergency number if it is not possible to safely or comfortably move the person to a vehicle for transport to a healthcare facility. While you are waiting for help to arrive, have the person rest in a position that will make breathing easier, monitor the person's breathing and give care for shock, if necessary.

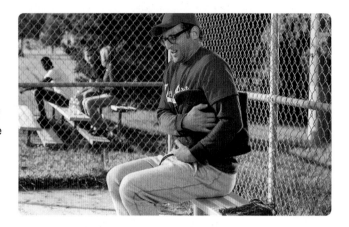

## Sucking Chest Wound

The care for a sucking chest wound is slightly different from the care for other types of open wounds. If external bleeding is present, apply direct pressure to the wound to control the bleeding, but remove each dressing as it becomes saturated with blood and replace it with a clean one as needed. If there is no external bleeding, do not cover the wound. It is important to avoid sealing an open chest wound because doing so could lead to life-threatening complications. While you are waiting for help to arrive, monitor the person's breathing and care for shock, if necessary.

# Abdominal Injuries

As with chest injuries, abdominal injuries can result from blunt or penetrating trauma and may be accompanied by internal bleeding. It is especially difficult to determine if a person has an abdominal injury if he or she is unresponsive and has no visible signs and symptoms of injury. Always suspect an abdominal injury in a person who has multiple injuries. Conversely, if a person has an abdominal injury, be sure to check the person for other injuries because abdominal injuries are often accompanied by injuries to the chest, pelvis or head.

## Signs and Symptoms of Abdominal Injuries

Signs and symptoms of a serious abdominal injury could include:

- Severe pain.
- Organs protruding from the abdomen.
- A tender, swollen or rigid abdomen.
- Bruising over the abdomen.
- Nausea.

- Vomiting (sometimes blood).
- Signs and symptoms of shock, such as excessive thirst; skin that feels cool or moist and looks pale or bluish; an altered level of consciousness; and a rapid, weak heartbeat.

# First Aid Care for Abdominal Injuries

Call 9-1-1 or the designated emergency number for any serious abdominal injury. Carefully position the person on his or her back with his or her knees bent, unless that position causes the person pain or the person has other injuries. While you are waiting for help to arrive, monitor the person's condition and give care for shock, if necessary.

Abdominal organs may protrude through a severe open wound. If organs are protruding through the wound, do not push them back in and do not apply direct pressure to try and stop minor bleeding. After putting on latex-free disposable gloves, remove clothing from around the wound. Moisten sterile dressings with clean, warm tap water or saline and apply them loosely over the wound. Then cover the dressings loosely with plastic wrap or aluminum foil, if available.

# Pelvic Injuries

The pelvis is a ring-shaped group of bones that provides support for the trunk; connects the trunk to the legs; and protects the bladder, the rectum, several major arteries and, in women, the reproductive organs. The hip joint is formed by the acetabulum (a cup-shaped indentation on the pelvis) and the upper part of the femur (the thigh bone).

Blunt trauma to the pelvic region can result in pelvic fractures and damage to the internal organs, blood vessels and nerves that are normally protected by the pelvic bones. Usually pelvic fractures result from high-energy impacts (for example, a motor-vehicle collision), but in older adults with osteoporosis (a disease in which loss of bone tissue causes the bones to become fragile and prone to breaking), minor trauma or a fall can result in breaking the pelvis or the upper part of the femur where it forms the hip joint with the pelvis. Pelvic injuries are serious and may be life threatening because of the risk of damage to major arteries or internal organs. Fractures of bones in this area may cause severe internal bleeding and are associated with an increased risk for death in older adults.

## Signs and Symptoms of Pelvic Injuries

Signs and symptoms of a pelvic injury may include the following:

- Severe pain at the site of the injury

- Bruising, swelling or both at the site of the injury

- Instability of the pelvic bones

- Blood-tinged urine

- Loss of sensation in the legs or an inability to move the legs

- Signs and symptoms of shock, such as excessive thirst; skin that feels cool or moist and looks pale or bluish; an altered level of consciousness; and a rapid, weak heartbeat

## First Aid Care for Pelvic Injuries

Always call 9-1-1 or the designated emergency number if you suspect a pelvic injury. Avoid moving the person unnecessarily because movement can make the pelvic injury worse, and the person may also have injuries to the lower spine. If possible, try to keep the person lying flat, and give care for shock if necessary.

# Using Direct Pressure to Control External Bleeding

1. Cover the wound with a sterile gauze pad and apply direct pressure until the bleeding stops.

   ■ If blood soaks through the first gauze pad, put another one on top and apply additional direct pressure (press harder than you did before, if possible). It may take several minutes for the bleeding to stop.

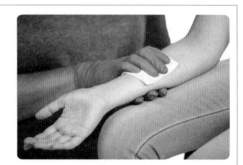

2. When the bleeding stops, check for circulation (feeling, warmth and color) beyond the injury.

3. Apply a roller bandage. Wrap the bandage around the wound several times to hold the gauze pad(s) in place.

   ■ Tie or tape the bandage to secure it.

   ■ Check for circulation (feeling, warmth and color) beyond the injury. If there is a change in feeling, warmth or color (indicating that the bandage is too tight), gently loosen it.

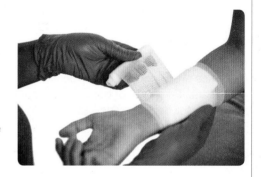

4. Remove your gloves and wash your hands.

**Note:** *If the bleeding does not stop with the application of direct pressure, call 9-1-1 or the designated emergency number if you have not already, and give care for shock if necessary.*

# Using a Commercial Tourniquet

**Note:** *Always follow the manufacturer's instructions when applying a tourniquet.*

1. Place the tourniquet around the limb, approximately 2 inches above the wound. Avoid placing the tourniquet over a joint.

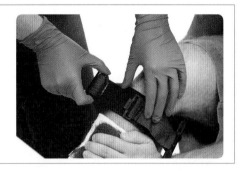

2. Secure the tourniquet tightly in place according to the manufacturer's instructions.

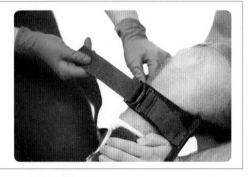

3. Tighten the tourniquet by twisting the rod until the flow of bright red blood stops.

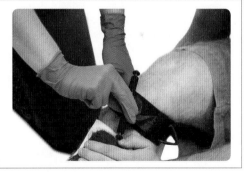

4. Secure the rod in place using the clip or holder.

5. Note and record the time that you applied the tourniquet and give this information to EMS personnel when they arrive.

   ■ Once you apply a tourniquet, do not loosen or remove it.

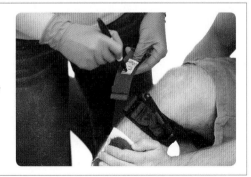

# 7 ENVIRONMENTAL INJURIES AND ILLNESSES

**A**lthough taking the proper precautions can lower risk for injury or illness caused by environmental factors, it is not possible to eliminate all environmental hazards, especially when work or play brings us outdoors. Weather conditions and chance interactions with the other living things that share our planet have the potential to create a first aid emergency. Knowing the signs and symptoms—especially the early ones—of environmentally caused illnesses and injuries will allow you to make quick decisions for yourself or others and could mean the difference between life and death.

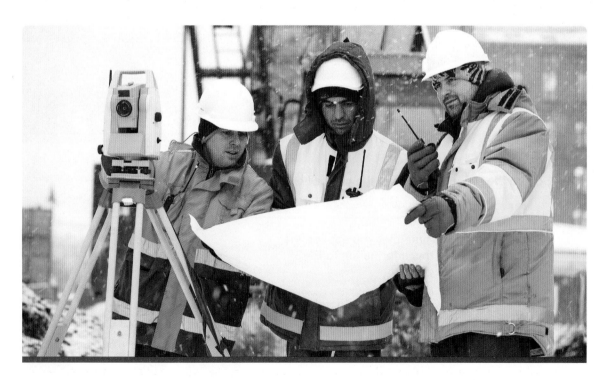

# Exposure Injuries and Illnesses

**Thermoregulation**, or the body's ability to maintain an internal temperature within an acceptable range despite external conditions, is important for human survival. The body uses various methods to achieve thermoregulation. For example, sweat evaporating from the skin helps to cool the body, and the muscle contractions caused by shivering help to warm the body. Usually the body is able to maintain a normal body temperature despite exposure to hot or cold external temperatures. However, under certain conditions (such as prolonged exposure to heat or cold, heavy exertion, inadequate fluid intake, or exposure to extreme heat or extreme cold), the body's thermoregulatory mechanisms can become overwhelmed, leading to life-threatening illness. People who are at increased risk for experiencing a first aid emergency due to exposure to heat or cold include:

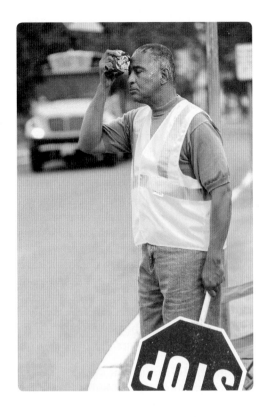

- Those who work or exercise outdoors.
- The elderly and the young.
- Those with medical conditions that cause poor blood circulation.
- Those who take diuretics (medications that promote the elimination of water from the body).

## Heat-Related Illnesses

Heat-related illnesses are caused by overexposure to heat and the loss of fluids and electrolytes. While being outdoors is a risk factor for developing a heat-related illness, these illnesses can also affect people who are indoors. People who live or work in buildings that are inadequately cooled or ventilated are at risk, as are those who perform indoor jobs in hot environments (e.g., kitchen and laundry workers, factory workers). People who habitually work or exercise in hot environments tend to become more tolerant of the heat over time but may still be at risk for developing heat-related illnesses, especially when environmental temperatures are very high (e.g., greater than 100° F or 38° C).

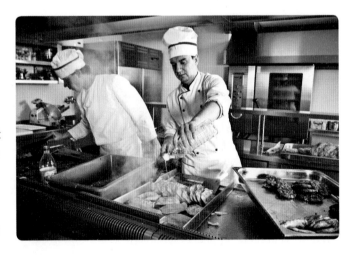

Although extremely high environmental temperatures increase the risk for heat-related illnesses, these illnesses can also occur at more moderate environmental temperatures. For example, a person who is doing strenuous work and is clothed in heavy protective clothing may be at risk for experiencing a heat-related illness at a lower environmental temperature. Similarly, a person who is unaccustomed to doing strenuous labor or exercising in the heat may develop a heat-related illness at lower environmental temperatures. Other factors, such as humid air, inadequate fluid intake and personal characteristics (e.g., the presence of certain medical conditions, the person's age) can increase the risk for heat-related illness.

The three types of heat-related illnesses (in order from least to most severe) are heat cramps, heat exhaustion and heat stroke.

# Heat Cramps

**Heat cramps** (painful muscle spasms, usually in the legs and abdomen, caused by loss of fluids and electrolytes as a result of sweating) are often the first sign that the body is having trouble with the heat. If appropriate care measures are not taken, heat cramps can turn into heat exhaustion or heat stroke. To care for heat cramps, help the person move to a cool place to rest, and have him or her sip a drink containing electrolytes and carbohydrates (such as a commercial sports drink, coconut water or milk). If a drink containing electrolytes and carbohydrates is not available, have the person drink water. Lightly stretch the muscle and gently massage the area to relieve the cramps. When the cramps stop, the person usually can resume his or her activity as long as there are no other signs or symptoms of illness. Encourage the person to keep drinking plenty of fluids, and watch the person carefully for additional signs or symptoms of heat-related illness.

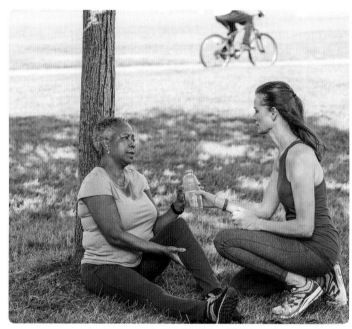

> **Myth-Information.** *Myth: When a person has heat cramps, you should give the person salt tablets to replenish lost sodium.* Salt tablets are not an effective treatment for heat cramps. Consuming a concentrated form of salt can promote loss of fluid from the body, which will make the person's condition worse, not better.

# Heat Exhaustion

**Heat exhaustion** occurs when fluids lost through sweating are not replaced. The body's primary mechanism of cooling itself is through sweating. As sweat evaporates from the body, it takes body heat with it, cooling the body. If a person does not take in enough fluids, the body does not have what it needs to make adequate amounts of sweat. Humid environments and environments without good air circulation can make it difficult for the sweat to evaporate. Under these conditions, a person may develop heat exhaustion. Heat exhaustion is often accompanied by dehydration, as the body's excessive production of sweat in an attempt to cool itself depletes fluid levels in the body.

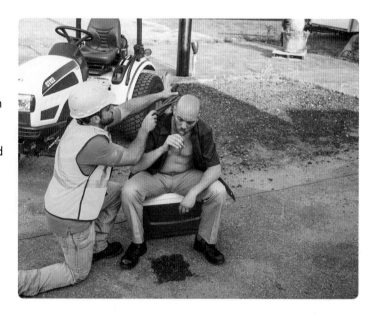

## Signs and Symptoms of Heat Exhaustion

The person's skin will be cool and moist, and pale, ashen (gray) or flushed. The person may complain of a headache, nausea, dizziness and weakness.

## First Aid Care for Heat Exhaustion

Move the person to a cooler environment with circulating air. Loosen or remove as much clothing as possible and apply cool, wet cloths to the person's skin or spray the person with cool water. Fanning the person may also help by increasing evaporative cooling. If the person is responsive and able to swallow, have the person drink a cool electrolyte- and carbohydrate-containing fluid (such as a commercial sports drink, coconut water or milk). Give water if none of these are available. Do not let the person drink too quickly. Encourage the person to rest in a comfortable position, and watch carefully for changes in his or her condition. Call 9-1-1 or the designated emergency number if the person's condition does not improve. The person should wait for several hours after he or she is no longer having signs and symptoms to resume activity.

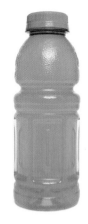

If the person is unable to take fluids by mouth, has a change in level of consciousness or vomits, call 9-1-1 or the designated emergency number, because these are indications that the person's condition is getting worse. Stop giving fluids and place the person in the recovery position. Keep the person lying down and continue to take steps to lower the person's body temperature. Monitor the person for signs and symptoms of breathing problems and shock.

## Heat Stroke

**Heat stroke** is the least common but most severe heat-related illness. It occurs when the body's cooling system is completely overwhelmed and stops working. Heat stroke is a life-threatening emergency.

### Signs and Symptoms of Heat Stroke

The person will have mental status changes (such as confusion or loss of consciousness) and may have trouble seeing or a seizure. The person's skin will be hot to the touch. It may be wet or dry and appear red or pale. The person may vomit. The person's breathing may be rapid and shallow, and his or her heartbeat may be rapid and weak.

### First Aid Care for Heat Stroke

Send someone to call 9-1-1 or the designated emergency number immediately. While you wait for help to arrive, take steps to rapidly cool the person's body. The preferred way of doing this is to immerse the person up to his or her neck in cold water, if you can do this safely. Alternatively, place ice water–soaked towels over the person's entire body, rotating the towels frequently. If bags of ice are available, place these on the person's body, over the towels. If you are not able to measure and monitor the person's temperature, apply rapid cooling methods for 20 minutes or until the person's condition improves or EMS personnel arrive. Give care as needed for other conditions that you find.

# Cold-Related Illnesses and Injuries

Exposure illnesses and injuries can also result from exposure to cold temperatures (Box 7-1).

## Hypothermia

In **hypothermia**, the body loses heat faster than it can produce heat, causing the core body temperature to fall below 95° F (35° C). Hypothermia can result from exposure to cold

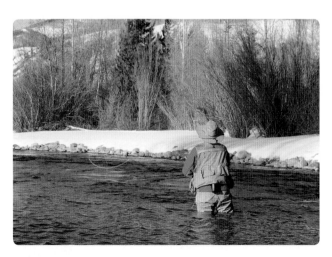

air or water temperatures, or both. Just as with heat-related illnesses, the air or water temperature does not have to be extreme (e.g., below freezing) for hypothermia to occur. Prolonged exposure to cold, wet or windy conditions and wet clothing increase risk for hypothermia, even at moderate environmental temperatures. As with heat-related illnesses, children and older adults are especially susceptible to hypothermia. Hypothermia can be fatal if the person does not receive prompt care.

## Signs and Symptoms of Hypothermia

A person who has hypothermia may seem indifferent, disoriented or confused. You may notice that the person has a "glassy" stare. Initially, the person may shiver, but as the hypothermia progresses, the shivering may stop. This is a sign that the person's condition is worsening and he or she needs immediate medical care. In advanced cases of hypothermia, the person may become unresponsive, and his or her breathing may slow or stop. The body may feel stiff because the muscles became rigid.

## Box 7-1. **Dressing for Cold Weather**

Dressing in layers can help to protect you from illness as a result of exposure to cold external temperatures.

The first layer, called the base layer, is next to your skin. The base layer helps to regulate your body temperature by wicking perspiration away from your skin. This is important because if perspiration gets trapped inside your clothes, you can become chilled rapidly, which can lead to hypothermia. The fabrics that are best at wicking sweat away from the skin are silk, merino wool and certain synthetics. Cotton is not a good choice because it traps moisture, rather than wicking it away.

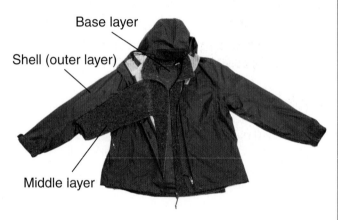

The job of the middle layer is insulation. This layer keeps you warm; it helps you retain heat by trapping air close to your body. Natural fibers, such as wool and goose down, are excellent insulators. So is synthetic fleece. Vests, jackets and tights are examples of clothing that can be worn for insulation.

The shell or outer layer protects you from wind, rain or snow. For cold weather, the shell layer should be both waterproof and "breathable." This will keep wind and water from getting inside of the other two layers while allowing perspiration to evaporate. The shell also should be roomy enough to fit easily over the other layers without restricting your movement.

In addition to layering your clothes, wear the following to stay warm in cold weather:

- A hat
- A scarf or knit mask that covers your face and mouth

- Sleeves that are snug at the wrist
- Mittens (they are warmer than gloves)
- Water-resistant boots

# First Aid Care for Hypothermia

Call 9-1-1 or the designated emergency number immediately for any case of hypothermia. If the person is unresponsive and not breathing or only gasping, give CPR and use an automated external defibrillator (AED) if you are trained in these skills.

Raising the body temperature must be accomplished gradually. Rapid rewarming (for example, by immersing the person in a hot bath or shower) can lead to dangerous heart rhythms and should be avoided. To gradually rewarm the person, gently move the person to a warm place. Remove any wet clothing, dry the person, and help the person to put on dry clothing (including a hat, gloves and socks). Then wrap the person in dry blankets and plastic sheeting, if available, to hold in body heat. If you are far from medical care, position the person near a heat source or apply heating pads or hot water bottles filled with warm water to the body. If you have positioned the person near a heat source, carefully monitor the heat source to avoid burning the person. If you are using heating pads or hot water bottles, wrap them in thin, dry cloths to protect the person's skin. If the person is alert and able to swallow, you can give the person small sips of a warm, non-caffeinated liquid such as broth or warm water. Continue warming the person and monitor the person for changes in condition (including changes in breathing or level of consciousness and the development of shock) until EMS personnel arrive.

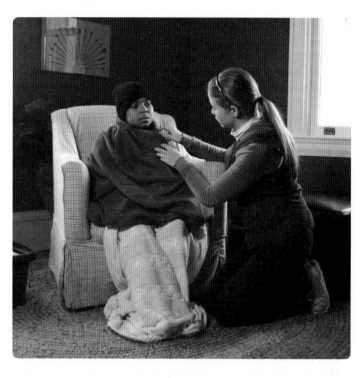

> **Myth-Information.** *Myth: Giving a person with hypothermia an alcoholic drink can help the person to warm up.* Never give alcohol to a person who has hypothermia. Although alcohol may temporarily make the person feel warmer, it actually increases loss of body heat. You should also avoid giving a person who has hypothermia beverages containing caffeine, because caffeine promotes fluid loss and can lead to dehydration.

# Frostbite

**Frostbite** is an injury caused by freezing of the skin and underlying tissues as a result of prolonged exposure to freezing or subfreezing temperatures. Frostbite can cause the loss of fingers, hands, arms, toes, feet and legs.

## Signs and Symptoms of Frostbite

The frostbitten area is numb, and the skin is cold to the touch and appears waxy. The skin may be white, yellow, blue or red. In severe cases, there may be blisters and the skin may turn black.

## First Aid Care for Frostbite

If the frostbite is severe or the person is also showing signs and symptoms of hypothermia, call 9-1-1 or the designated emergency number. Give care for hypothermia, if necessary. If the frostbite has caused blisters, do not break them. Monitor the person's condition, and if you see that the person is going into shock, give care accordingly.

If the frostbite is mild, you may be able to care for it using first aid. When providing first aid care for frostbite, handle the affected area gently. Never rub the frostbitten area, because this can cause additional damage to the tissue. Remove wet clothing and jewelry (if possible) from the affected area and care for hypothermia, if necessary.

Do not attempt to rewarm the frostbitten area if there is a chance that the body part could refreeze before the person receives medical attention. Once the rewarming process is started, the tissue cannot be allowed to refreeze because refreezing can lead to tissue necrosis (death). Skin-to-skin contact (for example, cupping the affected area in your hands) may be sufficient to rewarm the frostbitten body part if the frostbite is mild. Alternatively, you can rewarm the affected body part by soaking it in warm water until normal color and warmth returns (about 20 to 30 minutes). The water temperature should not be more than 100° F–105° F (38° C–40.5° C). If you do not have a thermometer, test the water with your hand. It should feel warm (about body temperature), not hot. After rewarming, loosely bandage the area with a dry, sterile bandage. If the fingers or toes were affected, place cotton or gauze between them before bandaging the area (Figure 7-1).

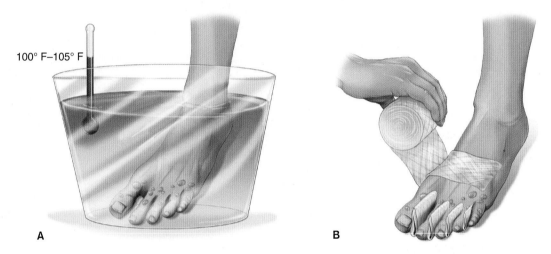

100° F–105° F

A                                    B

**Figure 7-1.** To care for frostbite, rewarm the body part by immersing it in warm water (A) and then loosely bandage it (B).

# Poisoning

A poison is any substance that causes injury, illness or death if it enters the body. Poisons can be ingested (swallowed), inhaled, absorbed through the skin or eyes, or injected. Practically anything can be a poison if it is not meant to be taken into the body. Even some substances that are meant to be taken into the body, such as medications, can be poisonous if they are taken by the wrong person, or if the person takes too much. Combining certain substances can also result in poisoning.

Poisoning can happen anywhere, but most poisonings take place in the home. Children younger than 5 years, especially toddlers, are at the highest risk for poisoning. Children may be attracted to pretty liquids in bottles, sweet-smelling powders, berries on plants that look like they are edible, or medications or vitamins that look like candy. Additionally, very young children explore their world by touching and tasting things around them, so even substances that do not look or smell attractive are poisoning hazards among this age group. Older adults who have medical conditions that cause confusion (such as dementia) or who have impaired vision are also at high risk for unintentional poisoning. Box 7-2 lists common household poisons, and Box 7-3 describes strategies for reducing the risk for unintentional poisoning at home.

Common causes of death as a result of poisoning include drug overdose (of over-the-counter, prescription and illicit or "street" drugs), alcohol poisoning and carbon monoxide poisoning (Box 7-4).

## Box 7-2. **Household Poisons**

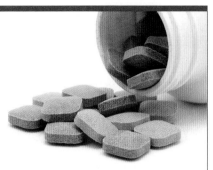

Many everyday household items can be poisonous if they are used incorrectly. Young children and older adults with medical conditions that are associated with confusion (e.g., dementia) or who have impaired vision are at particularly high risk for unintentional poisoning. Common causes of unintentional poisonings at home include:

- Alcohol (found in many products, including hand sanitizer, mouthwash, perfume, cologne, aftershave and vanilla extract).

- Medications (over-the-counter and prescription) and vitamins.

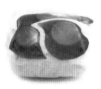

- Cleaning products (detergent "pods" are especially attractive to children).

- Glues and paints.

- Insect and weed killers.

- Car maintenance products (e.g., antifreeze, windshield washer fluid).

- Plants (both houseplants and outdoor plants).

- Oils, lubricants and polishes.

- Personal care products.

- Tobacco.

- Heavy metals, such as lead (often found in old, peeling paint).

## Box 7-3. **Lowering the Risk for Unintentional Poisoning**

If your household contains members who are at high risk for unintentional poisoning, there are simple steps you can take to help keep them safe:

- Keep all medications and household products well out of reach of children or confused older adults, preferably up, away and out of sight.

- Store potentially poisonous substances in locked cabinets.

- Be aware that purses and bags may contain potential poisons (such as medications or hand sanitizer). Avoid putting bags or purses down where they are within reach of curious children or confused older adults.

- Closely supervise children and confused older adults, especially in areas where potential poisons are commonly stored (such as kitchens, bathrooms and garages).

- Keep medications and products in their original containers with their original labels in place.

- Use poison symbols to identify potentially poisonous substances, and teach children the meaning of the symbols.

- Be aware that a child or confused older adult may try to consume products that feature fruit on the label (e.g., cleaning products), so take care when storing these.

- Never call a medicine "candy" to entice a child to take it, even if the medicine has a pleasant candy-like flavor.

- Use child-resistant safety caps on containers of medication and other potentially dangerous products, but do not assume that children cannot open them. (There is no such thing as "childproof.")

- Dispose of medications and other potentially poisonous substances properly. Check with your local government for procedures for the safe disposal of unused and expired medications and other hazardous materials.

# Box 7-4. **Lethal Poisons**

There are many different types of poisoning, but three in particular warrant special mention because they are common and often fatal: drug overdose, alcohol poisoning and carbon monoxide poisoning.

## Drug Overdose

Drugs (whether over-the-counter, prescription or illicit) are frequently a cause of death as a result of poisoning. Drug overdose may be accidental or intentional. Signs and symptoms will vary depending on the drug but may include loss of consciousness, changes in breathing and heart rate, and nausea or vomiting. If you suspect a drug overdose, call 9-1-1 or the designated emergency number if the person:

- Is unresponsive or seems to be losing consciousness.
- Is having difficulty breathing.
- Has persistent pain or pressure in the chest or abdomen.
- Is vomiting blood or passing blood.
- Has a seizure, severe headache or slurred speech.
- Is aggressive or uncooperative.

While you are waiting for EMS personnel to arrive, try to find out from others at the scene what substance or substances the person may have taken. Keep the person covered to minimize shock.

Opioid drugs, such as heroin and oxycodone, are a common cause of drug overdose in the United States. Signs and symptoms of opioid overdose include slowed breathing (or no breathing), extreme drowsiness or loss of consciousness, and small pupils. EMS personnel use naloxone (Narcan®) to reverse the effects of opioid drugs. In some states, lay responders can receive training in administering naloxone. For lay responder use, naloxone is supplied as a nasal spray.

## Alcohol Poisoning

Alcohol poisoning is caused by drinking large quantities of alcohol in a short period of time (binge drinking). The National Institute on Alcohol Abuse and Alcoholism defines binge drinking as a pattern of drinking that brings a person's blood alcohol concentration (BAC) to 0.08 percent or more. This typically happens when a man consumes 5 or more drinks over a period of about 2 hours, or when a woman consumes 4 or more drinks over the same amount of time. Alcohol is a depressant that affects the central nervous system. Very high levels of alcohol in the bloodstream can affect the brain's ability to control breathing, heart rate and body temperature, resulting in death. Signs and symptoms of alcohol poisoning include loss of consciousness, slow or irregular breathing, vomiting, seizures and hypothermia. If you suspect alcohol poisoning, call 9-1-1 or the designated emergency number immediately. Place the person in the recovery position and take steps to keep the airway clear as needed until EMS personnel arrive.

## Carbon Monoxide Poisoning

Carbon monoxide is a gas that is produced whenever a fuel such as gas, oil, kerosene, diesel, wood or charcoal is burned. When equipment that burns these fuels is ventilated properly, carbon monoxide is not a problem. But if the equipment or ventilation system is faulty, or if equipment that is only supposed to be run outdoors is run inside an enclosed area, toxic levels of carbon monoxide can build up quickly, leading to carbon monoxide poisoning. Carbon monoxide poisoning is often called a "silent killer" because the gas has no smell and you cannot see it. Signs and symptoms of carbon monoxide poisoning include drowsiness, confusion, headache, dizziness, weakness, and nausea or vomiting. A person with signs or symptoms of carbon monoxide poisoning needs fresh air and medical attention immediately. Remove the person from the area if you can do so without endangering yourself and call 9-1-1 or the designated emergency number.

# Signs and Symptoms of Poisoning

Signs and symptoms of poisoning vary depending on the type and amount of poison taken into the body. The person may experience:

- Gastrointestinal signs and symptoms, such as abdominal pain, nausea, vomiting or diarrhea.

- Respiratory signs and symptoms, such as difficulty breathing or slow and shallow breathing.

- Neurological signs and symptoms, such as changes in level of consciousness, seizures, headache, dizziness, weakness or irregular pupil size.

- Skin signs and symptoms, such as an unusual skin color or sweating.

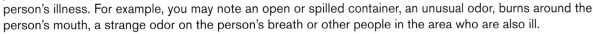

Your scene size-up and check of the person will often yield clues that point to poisoning as the cause of the person's illness. For example, you may note an open or spilled container, an unusual odor, burns around the person's mouth, a strange odor on the person's breath or other people in the area who are also ill.

If you think that a person has been poisoned, try to find out:

- The type of poison.

- The quantity taken.

- When it was taken.

- How much the person weighs.

This information can help you and others to give the most appropriate care.

# First Aid Care for Poisoning

If the person is showing signs and symptoms of a life-threatening condition (for example, loss of consciousness, difficulty breathing) or if multiple people are affected, call 9-1-1 or the designated emergency number.

If the person is responsive and alert, call the national Poison Help hotline at 1-800-222-1222. When you dial this number, your call is routed to the regional poison control center that serves your area, based on the area code and exchange of the phone number you are calling from (Box 7-5). The poison control center staff member will tell you what care to give. General first aid care steps for poisoning include the following:

- Remove the source of the poison if you can do so without endangering yourself.

- Do not give the person anything to eat or drink unless the poison control center staff member tells you to do so.

- If you do not know what the poison was and the person vomits, save a sample for analysis.

> **Myth-Information.** *Myth: If a person has been poisoned, you should make the person vomit to get rid of the poison.* Inducing vomiting in a person who has been poisoned often causes additional harm and is not recommended. Sometimes the person may vomit on his or her own, but you should never give the person anything to make him or her vomit unless you are specifically instructed to do so by the poison center staff member.

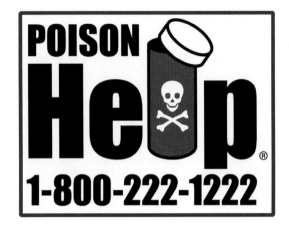
# Bites and Stings

Bites and stings can range in severity from mildly irritating to life threatening. When a person is bitten or stung, proper first aid care can help to limit complications and speed healing, and may even be lifesaving.

## Animal Bites

Any animal that has teeth, whether domesticated (e.g., pets or livestock) or wild, can be the source of a bite wound. When the animal is unknown to the person (e.g., a stray or wild animal), rabies may be a concern (Box 7-6).

### Signs and Symptoms of Animal Bites

Animal bites may result in bruising, breaks in the skin or both. Open wounds, such as the avulsion wounds and lacerations often caused by dog bites, may be accompanied by a great deal of bleeding. Puncture wounds, such as those often caused by cat bites, typically do not bleed as much.

### First Aid Care for Animal Bites

If the wound is deep or extensive, bleeding heavily or uncontrollably, or carries a high risk for infection (for example, a puncture wound), medical care will be needed. The person may need stitches, a tetanus booster shot or both. If the wound is bleeding heavily, take steps to control external bleeding and call 9-1-1 or the designated emergency number. You should also call 9-1-1 or the designated emergency number if the person was bitten by a wild or stray animal, or if you suspect that the animal might have rabies.

## Box 7-6. **Rabies**

Rabies is a serious infection that attacks the brain and spinal cord and causes death if it is not treated. The virus that causes rabies is spread when an animal that has the disease bites another animal or a person. Wild animals (such as foxes, skunks, bats and raccoons) can carry rabies. Pets and livestock can also carry rabies if they are not vaccinated against it.

Animals with rabies may act strangely. For example, those that are usually active at night may be active in the daytime. A wild animal that usually tries to avoid people might not run away when people are in the area. Rabid animals may drool, appear to be partially paralyzed, or act aggressively or strangely quiet.

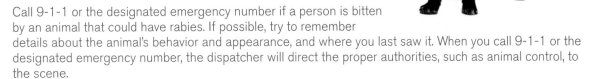

Call 9-1-1 or the designated emergency number if a person is bitten by an animal that could have rabies. If possible, try to remember details about the animal's behavior and appearance, and where you last saw it. When you call 9-1-1 or the designated emergency number, the dispatcher will direct the proper authorities, such as animal control, to the scene.

A person who is bitten by an animal that might have rabies must get medical attention immediately. Treatment for rabies includes a series of injections to build up immunity that will help fight the disease.

---

If the bleeding is minimal, wash the wound with soap and water and then rinse with clean, running water. Apply a small amount of antibiotic wound ointment, cream or gel to the wound if the person has no known allergies or sensitivities to the ingredients, and then cover the wound with a dressing and bandage. The person should monitor the wound over the next several days to make sure that it is healing well with no signs of infection (see Chapter 6, Box 6-1).

# Venomous Snake Bites

Venomous snakes found in the United States include rattlesnakes, copperheads, cottonmouths (water moccasins) and coral snakes (Table 7-1). Prompt medical care significantly reduces the likelihood of dying from a venomous snake bite. Most deaths from venomous snake bites occur because the person had an allergic reaction to the venom or is in poor health, or because too much time passed before he or she received medical care.

## Signs and Symptoms of Venomous Snake Bites

Signs and symptoms of a possibly venomous snakebite include a pair of puncture wounds and localized redness, pain and swelling in the area of the bite.

## First Aid Care for Venomous Snake Bites

Call 9-1-1 or the designated emergency number immediately. If you are not sure whether the snake bite was caused by a venomous snake, call 9-1-1 or the designated emergency number anyway. Do not waste time trying to find and capture the snake for identification, and do not wait for life-threatening signs and symptoms of poisoning to appear.

## TABLE 7-1 Venomous Snakes

| Snake | Usually Found |
|---|---|
| **Rattlesnake**<br> | ■ Across the United States<br><br>■ Mountains, prairies, deserts and beaches<br><br>■ Sunning themselves near logs, boulders or in open areas |
| **Copperhead**<br> | ■ Eastern United States, extending as far west as Texas<br><br>■ Forests, rocky areas and near sources of water like swamps and rivers |
| **Cottonmouth (water moccasin)**<br> | ■ Southeastern United States<br><br>■ Frequently found in and around water (wetland areas, rivers and lakes) |
| **Coral snake**<br><br>To differentiate coral snakes from nonvenomous king snakes, which have similar coloration but in a different pattern, think "Red on yellow, dangerous fellow." | ■ Southern United States<br><br>■ Wooded, sandy or marshy areas<br><br>■ Tend to hide in leaf piles and burrow into the ground |

Keep the injured area still and lower than the heart. The person should walk only if absolutely necessary. Wash the wound with soap and water; cover the bite with a clean, dry dressing; and then apply an elastic (pressure immobilization) bandage to slow the spread of the venom through the lymphatic system, to control swelling and to provide support. To apply an elastic bandage:

- Check the skin on the side of the bite farthest away from the heart for feeling, warmth and color.

- Place the end of the bandage against the skin, beginning at the point farthest from the heart.

- To cover a long body section, such as an arm or calf, use overlapping turns and gently stretch the bandage as you wrap. To cover a joint, such as the knee or ankle, use overlapping figure-eight turns to support the joint (Figure 7-2).

- Check the snugness of the bandage—it should be snug but you should be able to slide a finger easily underneath it.

- Check again for feeling, warmth and color, especially in the fingers and toes, after you have applied the elastic bandage. By checking before and after bandaging, you may be able to tell if any changes (e.g., tingling or numbness, cool or pale skin) are from the elastic bandage or the injury.

> **Myth-Information.** *Myth: Actions such as applying a tourniquet, cutting the wound, applying suction, applying ice or applying electricity can help to slow the spread of venom throughout the body.* None of these measures are effective for slowing the spread of venom. In fact, they are likely to cause pain and injury. Your time is better spent seeking medical attention as quickly as possible.

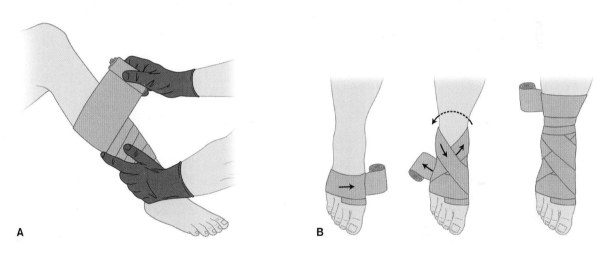

A          B

**Figure 7-2.** To apply a pressure immobilization bandage over a long body section, use overlapping turns and gently stretch the bandage as you wrap (A). To cover a joint, use overlapping figure-eight turns (B).

# Spider Bites

Few spiders in the United States can cause serious illness or death. The bites of harmless spiders cause reactions similar to that of a bee sting (e.g., swelling, redness, and stinging or pain at the site).

Dangerous spiders that live in the United States include the brown recluse spider (also known as the violin or fiddleback spider) and the black widow spider (Table 7-2). The bites of the black widow and brown recluse spiders can, in rare cases, kill a person.

## Signs and Symptoms of Spider Bites

Signs and symptoms of spider bites depend on the amount of venom injected and the person's sensitivity to the venom. Most spider bites heal with no adverse effects or scarring. Signs and symptoms of venomous spider bites can seem identical to those of other conditions and therefore can be difficult to recognize. The only way to be certain that a spider has bitten a person is to have witnessed it.

## TABLE 7-2 Venomous Spiders

| Spider | Usually Found |
|---|---|
| Black widow spider | ■ Across the United States, but most common in the southern states<br><br>■ Outdoors: woodpiles, rockpiles, brush piles, hollow stumps, rodent burrows, sheds and garages<br><br>■ Indoors: cluttered, undisturbed areas in attics, basements and crawlspaces |
| Brown recluse spider | ■ Midwestern and southeastern United States<br><br>■ Under porches and in woodpiles |

## Widow Spiders

Widow spiders can be black, red or brown. The black widow spider is black with a reddish hourglass shape on the underside of its body and is the most venomous of the widow spiders. The bite of the black widow spider is the most painful and deadly of the widow spiders, especially in very young children and older adults. The bite usually causes an immediate sharp pinprick pain, followed by dull pain in the area of the bite. However, the person often does not know that he or she has been bitten until he or she starts to feel ill or notices a bite mark or swelling. Other signs and symptoms of a black widow spider bite include:

- Rigid muscles in the shoulders, chest, back and abdomen.
- Restlessness.
- Anxiety.
- Dizziness.
- Headache.
- Excessive sweating.
- Weakness.
- Drooping or swelling of the eyelids.

## Brown Recluse Spiders

The brown recluse spider has a distinctive violin-shaped pattern on the back of its front body section. The bite of the brown recluse spider may produce little or no pain initially. Pain in the area of the bite develops an hour or more later. A blood-filled blister forms under the surface of the skin, sometimes in a target or bull's-eye pattern. Over time, the blister increases in size and eventually ruptures, leading to tissue destruction and a black scab.

## First Aid Care for Spider Bites

To care for a spider bite from a harmless spider, wash the area with soap and water; apply an antibiotic wound ointment, cream or gel to the wound if the person has no known allergies or sensitivities to the ingredients; and then cover the wound with an adhesive bandage. Applying a cold pack wrapped in a thin, dry towel can help to reduce pain and swelling.

If you suspect that someone has been bitten by a black widow spider or brown recluse spider, wash the area with soap and water. Apply a cold pack wrapped in a thin, dry towel; keep the bitten area elevated and as still as possible; and seek medical attention.

# Tick Bites

Ticks attach themselves to any warm-blooded animal with which they come into direct contact, including people. When ticks attach themselves to the skin, they can spread pathogens from their mouths into the person's body. These pathogens can cause serious illnesses, such as Lyme disease and Rocky Mountain spotted fever. Box 7-7 describes strategies for limiting exposure to ticks.

To lower the risk for tick-borne illnesses, always check for ticks immediately after outdoor activities. Most experts believe that the longer the tick stays attached to the skin, the greater the chances are of infection, so it is a good practice to check for ticks at least once daily after having been outdoors. Promptly remove any ticks that you find before they become swollen with blood.

To remove a tick, put on gloves. Using fine-tipped, pointed tweezers with a smooth inside surface, grasp the tick at the head as close to the skin as possible. Pull upward slowly and steadily without twisting until the tick releases its hold (Figure 7-3). Seal the tick in a container to help the healthcare provider with identifying the type of tick later. Wash the area with soap and warm water and then apply an antibiotic wound ointment, cream or gel if the person has no known allergies or sensitivities to the ingredients. If you are unable to remove the tick, or if you think that the tick's mouth parts are still embedded in the skin, the person should see a healthcare provider.

> **Myth-Information.** *Myth: To remove a tick, burn it off with a match or smother it with petroleum jelly or nail polish.* These folk remedies are not the best way to go about removing a tick. They rely on the tick detaching itself, which could take hours. As long as the tick's mouth parts are in contact with the skin, the tick is potentially transmitting disease. The goal is to remove the tick in one piece as quickly as possible. The best tool for doing this is a pair of fine-tipped tweezers or a special tick removal tool, such as a tick key.

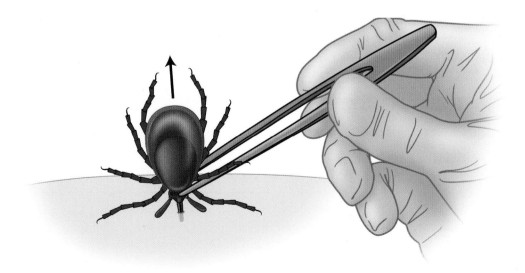

**Figure 7-3. Grasp the tick's head and pull straight up.**

The person should be monitored for several days for signs and symptoms of infection as a result of the tick exposure. Common signs and symptoms of tick-borne illnesses include rashes, fever, muscle and joint aches and pains, and fatigue.

---

## Box 7-7. **Lowering the Risk for Tick-Borne Illnesses**

Ticks are found in wooded, brushy areas; in tall grass; and in leaf litter on the ground. When engaging in activities in environments where ticks are likely to be, lower your risk for picking up a tick by using the following strategies:

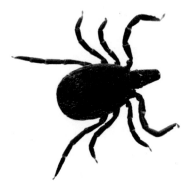

■ Limit the amount of exposed skin. Wear long-sleeved shirts and long pants. Tuck your shirt into your pants and your pant legs into your socks or boots.

■ Wear light-colored clothing to make it easier to see ticks on your clothing.

■ Stay in the middle of trails. Avoid underbrush and tall grass.

■ Conduct a full-body check for ticks after being outdoors.
Check the scalp, under the arms, in and around the ears, inside the navel, around the waist, behind the knees and between the legs. If you are outdoors for an extended period of time, check several times throughout the day.

■ Consider using an insect repellent if you will be in a grassy or wooded area for a long period of time or if you know that the tick population in the area is high. Use repellents sparingly. One application will last 4 to 8 hours. Heavier or more frequent applications do not increase effectiveness.

  ○ DEET is the active ingredient in many insect repellents. The amount of DEET contained in the product can range from less than 10 percent to over 30 percent. The more DEET that a product contains, the longer it will provide protection. Products with 30 percent DEET are as safe as products with 10 percent DEET when used properly.

    ■ Apply products that contain DEET only once a day, or according to the manufacturer's instructions.

    ■ Do not use DEET on infants younger than 2 months.

    ■ Do not use a product that combines a DEET-containing insect repellent with sunscreen. Sunscreens wash off and need to be reapplied often. DEET does not wash off with water. Repeating applications may increase absorption of DEET through the skin, possibly leading to toxicity.

  ○ To apply repellent to your face, first spray it on your hands and then apply it from your hands to your face. Avoid sensitive areas such as the lips and eyes.

  ○ Never put repellents on children's hands. They may put them in their eyes or mouth.

  ○ Never use repellents on an open wound or irritated skin.

# Insect Stings

Most of the time, insect stings are merely uncomfortable. However, allergic reactions and anaphylaxis are always a concern.

## Signs and Symptoms of Insect Stings

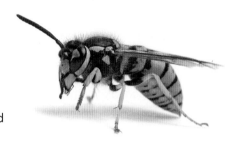

Signs and symptoms of an insect sting include a quick, sharp pain at the site of the sting, often accompanied by pain, itching, swelling and redness. You may see the stinger still embedded in the skin. If the person is allergic to insect stings, the person will show signs and symptoms of an allergic reaction or anaphylaxis (see Chapter 5).

## First Aid Care for Insect Stings

If the person is showing signs and symptoms of anaphylaxis, call 9-1-1 or the designated emergency number immediately and provide appropriate first aid care while you wait for help to arrive (see Chapter 5).

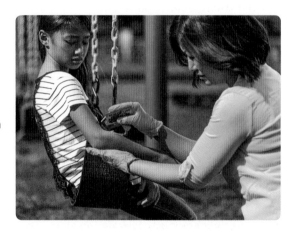

For an uncomplicated insect sting, use a plastic card (such as a credit card) to scrape the stinger away from the skin. Wash the area with soap and warm water and then apply an antibiotic wound ointment, cream or gel if the person has no known allergies or sensitivities to the ingredients. Cover the site with an adhesive bandage. To reduce swelling and pain, apply a cold pack wrapped in a thin, dry towel to the site.

# Scorpion Stings

Scorpions live in dry regions, such as the southwestern United States and Mexico. They live under rocks, logs and the bark of certain trees. They are most active at night. Like spiders, only a few species of scorpions have a sting that can cause death.

## Signs and Symptoms of Scorpion Stings

A scorpion sting causes pain, tingling, burning and numbness at the site. Life-threatening signs and symptoms that affect the whole body (such as numbness, difficulty breathing and seizures) may develop.

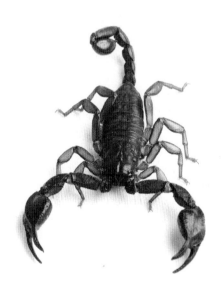

## First Aid Care For Scorpion Stings

It is difficult to distinguish highly poisonous scorpions from nonpoisonous scorpions, so treat every scorpion sting as a medical emergency and seek immediate medical care.

# Marine Life Stings

Many forms of marine life (such as jellyfish, stingrays, sea urchins, stinging coral and spiny fish) cause stinging wounds (Table 7-3). Stings from marine life can have effects that range from merely painful to very serious (such as allergic reactions that can cause breathing and heart problems, paralysis or even death).

## Signs and Symptoms of Marine Life Stings

Signs and symptoms of marine life stings include pain and swelling at the site. You may also see a puncture wound or laceration. If the person is allergic to marine life stings, the person will show signs and symptoms of an allergic reaction or anaphylaxis (see Chapter 5).

## First Aid Care for Marine Life Stings

Call 9-1-1 or the designated emergency number if the person has been stung by a lethal jellyfish, does not know what stung him or her, has a history of allergic reactions to marine life stings, is stung on the face or neck, or starts to have trouble breathing.

### Jellyfish Stings

Get the person out of the water as soon as possible, then take steps to neutralize the toxin and reduce pain. For most types of jellyfish typically found along the east and west coasts of the United States, flush the injured area with vinegar for at least 30 seconds to offset the toxin. You can also apply a baking soda slurry if vinegar is not available. For Portuguese man-of-war (bluebottle jellyfish), which are found in tropical waters, flush with ocean water instead of vinegar. Do not flush any jellyfish sting with fresh water, ammonia or rubbing alcohol because these substances may increase pain. Carefully remove any stingers or tentacles with gloved hands or a towel. After deactivating or removing the stingers or tentacles, immerse the affected area in water as hot as the person can tolerate (no more than about 113° F [45° C] if the temperature can be measured) for at least 20 minutes or until the pain is relieved. If hot water is not available, use dry hot packs, or as a second choice, dry cold packs to help decrease the pain. (Remember to wrap the hot or cold packs in a thin, dry towel to protect the skin.) Do not rub the area or apply an elastic (pressure immobilization) bandage.

### Stingray, Sea Urchin or Spiny Fish Stings

If you know the sting is from a stingray, sea urchin or spiny fish, flush the wound with tap water. Ocean water also may be used. Keep the injured part still and soak the affected area in water as hot as the person can tolerate for at least 20 minutes or until the pain is relieved. Check with a healthcare provider to determine if a tetanus shot is needed and monitor the wound for signs and symptoms of infection.

# Rash-Causing Plants

Plants such as poison ivy, poison sumac and poison oak (Table 7-4) are covered with an oil called **urushiol** that causes an allergic skin reaction in many people. In people who are sensitive to urushiol, touching or brushing against the plant or other items contaminated with urushiol causes an itchy, red rash with bumps or blisters. The rash can range from irritating to incapacitating, depending on the person's sensitivity, the amount of exposure and the rash's location. If urushiol is inhaled via smoke caused by burning the plants, severe reactions can result, including irritation of the lungs and swelling of the throat.

**TABLE 7-3** Venomous Marine Life

| Marine Life | Usually Found |
|---|---|
| Jellyfish | ■ East and west coasts of the continental United States |
| Portuguese man-of-war (bluebottle jellyfish) | ■ Tropical and subtropical waters |
| Stingray | ■ Tropical and subtropical waters |
| Sea urchin | ■ Oceans all over the world (warm and cold water)<br>■ In rock pools and mud, on wave-exposed rocks, on coral reefs, in kelp forests and in sea grass beds |

**TABLE 7-4** Rash-Causing Plants

| Plant | Usually Found |
|---|---|
| Poison ivy 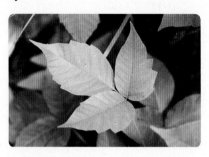 | ■ Throughout the United States, except for California, Alaska and Hawaii |
| Poison oak 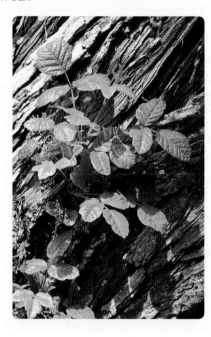 | ■ Southeastern United States and along the west coast |
| Poison sumac 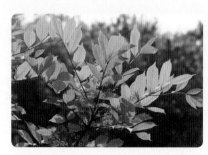 | ■ Eastern and southeastern United States (especially prevalent along the Mississippi River and in boggy areas of the southeast)<br><br>■ Texas |

Prevention is the best strategy. Although "leaves of three, let it be" is a good guideline for identifying poison ivy and poison oak, rash-causing plants vary in appearance depending on the species and time of year. It is a good idea to familiarize yourself with the appearance of the rash-causing plants in your area. If you will be engaging in activities where you could potentially be exposed to a rash-causing plant, wear a long-sleeved shirt, long pants and boots. Applying a pre-contact barrier cream or lotion before you go outside can help prevent urushiol from contacting your skin and causing a rash. Similarly, washing with a specialized skin cleanser designed to remove urushiol or a degreasing soap (such as dishwashing liquid) and plenty of water as soon as soon as you come in from outside can remove the urushiol from your skin and may prevent a rash from developing, or minimize the severity of the rash if one does develop. Wash tools, work gloves and clothing too because urushiol can remain on these surfaces and transfer to your skin the next time you use the item.

If exposure does result in a rash, apply calamine lotion or hydrocortisone cream to the area to reduce itching and blistering. An oral antihistamine may also help to relieve itching. If the rash is severe or on a sensitive part of the body (such as the face or groin), the person should see a healthcare provider. Call 9-1-1 or the designated emergency number if the person experiences a severe allergic reaction or is having trouble breathing.

# Lightning-Strike Injuries

Lightning travels at speeds of up to 300 miles per second. Anything tall—a tower, tree or person—can become a path for the electrical current (Box 7-8). Lightning can "flash" over a person's body or it can travel through blood vessels and nerves to reach the ground. The electrical energy can cause burn injuries and cardiac arrest. When the force of the lightning strike is sufficient to throw the person through the air, traumatic injuries such as fractures or dislocations can result.

## Signs and Symptoms of Lightning-Strike Injuries

A person who has been struck by lightning may seem dazed and confused, or he or she may be unresponsive. The person may be having difficulty breathing, or he or she may not be breathing at all. The person may have burn injuries; open wounds; or muscle, bone or joint injuries.

## First Aid Care for Lightning-Strike Injuries

Call 9-1-1 or the designated emergency number immediately if a person is struck by lightning. If the person is unresponsive and not breathing or only gasping, give CPR and use an AED if you are trained in these skills. Provide care for any other conditions that you find, such as burns; muscle, bone or joint injuries; or shock. Even if the person does not seem to have serious injuries and quickly recovers after the incident, he or she should still see a healthcare provider for follow-up evaluation and care.

## Box 7-8. **Avoiding Lightning-Strike Injuries**

Taking cover is the best strategy for preventing lightning-strike injuries. If you are outdoors, seek cover in a substantial building or a fully enclosed vehicle at the first sound of thunder or sight of lightning, even if it is not raining. Remember the 30/30 rule: take cover when the time between a flash of lightning and a roll of thunder is 30 seconds or less, and remain under cover until 30 minutes after the last flash of lightning was seen or the last roll of thunder was heard. If you are outside and cannot reach safety inside of a building, look for a low area. Avoid high ground, tall trees that stand alone, wide-open spaces (such as meadows) and structures such as sheds, dugouts, bleachers and picnic pavilions. These areas are not safe in a thunderstorm.

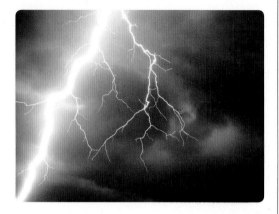

If no safe shelter is available, squat with your feet together and your arms wrapped around your legs. Stay low but do not lie flat. The less of your body that is in contact with the ground, the better.

# APPENDIX A

# EMERGENCY MOVES

Generally speaking, you should avoid moving an injured or ill person to give care. Unnecessary movement can cause additional injury and pain and may complicate the person's recovery. However, under the following three conditions, it would be appropriate to move an injured or ill person:

- You must move the person to protect him or her from immediate danger (such as fire, flood or poisonous gas). However, you should only attempt this if you can reach the person and remove him or her from the area without endangering yourself.

- You must move the person to reach another person who may have a more serious injury or illness.

- You must move the person to give proper care. For example, it may be necessary to move a person who needs CPR onto a hard, flat surface.

If you must move a person in an emergency situation, the goal is to do so without injuring yourself or causing additional injury to the person. The following common emergency moves can be done by one or two people and with minimal or no equipment. The situation will dictate which move you should use.

| Move | When to Use It | How to Do It |
|---|---|---|
| **Walking Assist**<br> | To move a person who can walk but needs help* | 1. Place the person's arm around your shoulder or waist (depending on how tall the person is), and hold it in place with one hand.<br><br>2. Support the person with your other hand around the person's waist.<br><br>(Another responder can also support the person in the same way on the other side.) |

| Move | When to Use It | How to Do It |
|---|---|---|
| **Two-Person Seat Carry** 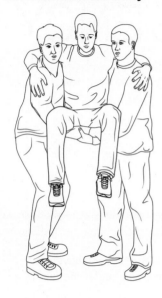 | To move a responsive person who is not seriously injured* | 1. Put one arm under the person's thighs and the other across his or her back, under his or her arms. Have a second responder do the same.<br><br>2. Interlock your arms with the other responder's arms under the person's legs and across the person's back.<br><br>3. Lift the person in the "seat" formed by your interlocked arms. |
| **Clothes Drag** 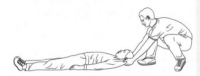 | To move a responsive or unresponsive person who may have a head, neck or back injury | 1. Grasp the person's shirt behind the neck, gathering enough material so that you have a firm grip.<br><br>2. Cradle the person's head with the shirt and your hands, and pull the person to safety. |
| **Blanket Drag** 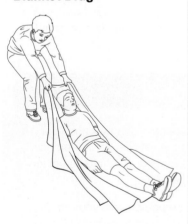 | To move a responsive or unresponsive person | 1. Fold the blanket in half lengthwise, and place it so that the fold is alongside the person's body.<br><br>2. Take the top layer of the folded blanket, and roll it toward the person's body.<br><br>3. Position yourself so that the person is between you and the blanket.<br><br>4. Put one hand on the person's shoulder and the other on his hip and roll the person onto his or her side, toward you, and then pull the blanket toward you so that it is against the person's body.<br><br>5. Roll the person onto his or her back, onto the blanket.<br><br>6. Pull the side of the blanket that was rolled up toward yourself, so that the person is in the middle of the blanket.<br><br>7. Gather the blanket at the person's head and pull the person to safety. |

| Move | When to Use It | How to Do It |
|---|---|---|
| **Ankle Drag** | To move a person who is too large to move another way | 1. Cross the person's arms over his or her chest.<br><br>2. Firmly grasp the person's ankles.<br><br>3. Move backward, pulling the person in a straight line and being careful not to bump the person's head. |

*Do not use this emergency move if you suspect that the person has a head, neck or spinal injury.

# APPENDIX

# SPECIAL FIRST AID SITUATIONS

## Abuse

**Abuse** is the willful infliction of injury or harm on another. People who depend on others for care, such as children and the elderly, are at the highest risk for being abused. Abuse can take many forms, including physical abuse (deliberately hurting another person's body), emotional abuse (degrading, belittling or threatening another person), sexual abuse (forcing a person to take part in sexual activities of any kind) and neglect (failing to provide for a dependent person's basic needs).

Signs and symptoms of abuse could include:

- An injury whose cause does not fit its explanation.

- Unexplained fractures or dislocations.

- Unexplained lacerations or abrasions, especially to the mouth, lips and eyes.

- Injuries in various stages of healing, especially bruises and burns.

- Bruises and burns in unusual shapes, such as bruises shaped like belt buckles or handprints, or burns the size of a cigarette tip.

- Bruises, scratches or cuts around the breasts, buttocks or genitals.

- A withdrawn or fearful demeanor, especially in the presence of the person who is causing the abuse.

Signs and symptoms of neglect could include:

- Lack of appropriate supervision.

- Signs of poor personal hygiene.

- Signs of dehydration.

- Signs of malnutrition.

- An unsafe living environment.

- Untreated chronic illness (e.g., a person with asthma who has no medications).

In a first aid situation, you may have reason to suspect that the person is a victim of abuse. Your priority is to give first aid care for the person's injury or illness, according to the conditions that you find and your level of training. If you suspect abuse, share your concerns with the responding emergency medical services (EMS) personnel, if possible. You can also report your suspicions to a community or state agency, such as the Department of Social Services, the Department of Child and Family Services, Child Protective Services, or Adult Protective Services.

You may be hesitant to report suspected abuse because you do not wish to get involved or are concerned about legal action. In most states, when you make a report in good faith, you are protected from any civil or criminal liability or penalty, even if the report was made in error. In this instance, good faith means that you honestly believe that abuse has occurred or the potential for abuse exists, and that a prudent and reasonable person in the same position would also honestly believe that abuse has occurred or the potential for abuse exists. You do not need to identify yourself when you report abuse, although your report will have more credibility if you do. In some professions (e.g., daycare or healthcare), employees are legally obligated to report suspicions of abuse of a person in their care to their supervisor (or to another person in the organization, per their employer's policy).

# Emergency Childbirth

Most women plan to deliver their babies with healthcare providers in attendance, either at the hospital or at home. But sometimes babies do not follow the plan and arrive unexpectedly and quickly. You may find yourself in the position of helping a woman to deliver a baby. Keep in mind that childbirth is a natural process and the body knows what to do. Your primary role will be to provide comfort and reassurance and to facilitate the process while you wait for help to arrive. Remember, the woman delivers the baby, so be patient and let it happen naturally.

A woman who is about to give birth will be experiencing regular contractions that are about 1 to 2 minutes apart. She may feel the urge to bear down or like she needs to have a bowel movement. The baby's head may be visible at the opening of the vagina (crowning).

Call 9-1-1 or the designated emergency number immediately. Be prepared to tell the EMS dispatcher the woman's age and expected due date, how long the woman has been having contractions, the time between contractions and how long each contraction is lasting, and whether or not this is the woman's first child.

The labor and delivery process will happen without much intervention on your part. Perhaps as important as what you should do is what you should *not* do:

- Do not let the woman leave to use the restroom. (The woman could deliver the baby into the toilet, putting the baby at risk for injury.)

- Do not try to delay delivery (for example, by holding the woman's legs together or trying to push the baby back into the vagina). This can cause serious injuries to both the mother and the baby.

- Do not place your fingers in the woman's vagina for any reason. This can introduce pathogens that can cause an infection.

- Do not pull on the baby.

Provide reassurance, privacy and comfort. Put someone in charge of clearing the area of unnecessary bystanders, and put on appropriate personal protective equipment (PPE), including gloves, a gown, a mask and eye protection if available. Position the woman on her back with her knees bent, feet flat and legs spread wide apart. Place several layers of clean padding (e.g., sheets, blankets or towels) under the woman's buttocks. Place an additional clean sheet, towel or blanket over the woman's abdomen. Be prepared to support the baby's head as it emerges. When the baby arrives, use a clean towel to receive and hold him or her. Handle the baby carefully because he or she will be slippery. Place the baby on the mother's stomach. If possible, note and record the time of birth. Do not cut the umbilical cord. If the placenta is delivered before EMS personnel arrive, handle it as little as possible. Carefully wrap it and save it for EMS personnel to take to the hospital along with the mother and baby.

# SPECIAL CONSIDERATIONS FOR SIGNS AND SYMPTOMS IN CHILDREN

## Fever

Fever is defined as an elevated body temperature above the normal range of 97.7° F–99.5° F (36.5° C–37.5° C). Fever is a common sign of illness in children and is often accompanied by other signs and symptoms of illness, such as a headache, muscle aches, chills, loss of appetite, low energy, difficulty sleeping and vomiting. An infant who has a fever may seem fussy, or he or she may be quiet and not as active as usual.

Fevers that last a long time or are very high can result in febrile seizures. A **febrile seizure** is a convulsion brought on by a fever in an infant or small child. Febrile seizures are the most common types of seizures in children. Most febrile seizures last less than 5 minutes and are not life threatening. Call 9-1-1 or the designated emergency number for a febrile seizure if:

■ This is the first time that a child has had a febrile seizure.

■ The seizure lasts longer than 5 minutes or is repeated.

■ The seizure is followed by a quick increase in body temperature.

When a child or infant has a fever, make him or her as comfortable as possible and encourage the child to rest. Check to ensure that the child or infant is not overdressed or covered with too many blankets. Usually a single layer of clothing and a light blanket is all that is necessary. As long as the child or infant is alert and able to swallow, offer clear liquids such as water, juice or chicken broth, or continue to nurse or bottle-feed to prevent dehydration.

If the child has a high fever, it is important to gently cool the child. Never rush cooling down a child. If the fever has caused a febrile seizure, rapid cooling could bring on other complications. Instead, remove any excessive clothing or blankets and sponge the child with lukewarm water.

> **Myth-Information.** *Rubbing alcohol helps cool the body and bring down a fever.* Rubbing alcohol (isopropyl alcohol) is dangerous to use to bring down a fever. It is quickly absorbed through the skin and is easily inhaled, placing the infant or child at risk for alcohol poisoning. Moreover, alcohol only cools the skin; it does not lower the internal body temperature.

**THE PROS KNOW.**
———

Never give aspirin to an infant or child who has a fever or other signs or symptoms of a flu-like or other viral illness. In this situation, taking aspirin can result in Reye's syndrome, an extremely serious and life-threatening condition that causes swelling in the brain and liver.

Contact a healthcare provider if:

- The infant is younger than 3 months and has a fever of 100.4° F or greater.

- The child is younger than 2 years and has a fever of 103° F or greater.

- The child or infant has a febrile seizure.

# Vomiting and Diarrhea

Vomiting, diarrhea or both are frequently signs and symptoms of infection in children. In young children, vomiting, diarrhea or both can lead to **dehydration** (too little fluid in the body) and shock. Infants and young children are at especially high risk for dehydration because they tend to lose more fluid, and at a faster rate, than adults do.

When a child or infant has an illness that causes vomiting, replace solid foods with clear fluids (e.g., water, popsicles, gelatin or oral rehydration solutions designed specifically for children and infants) for 24 hours. Wait 2 to 3 hours after a vomiting episode to offer the infant or child fluids. Offer 1 to 2 ounces every half hour, four times. Then alternate 2 ounces of rehydration solution with 2 ounces of water every 2 hours. After 12 to 24 hours with no vomiting, gradually reintroduce the infant's or child's normal diet.

To care for diarrhea:

- Maintain the infant's or child's normal well-balanced diet, including a mix of fruits, vegetables, meat, yogurt and complex carbohydrates. Try to limit sugar and artificial sweeteners.

- If the infant will not tolerate his or her normal feedings, or if the child is drinking less fluid than usual, add a commercially available oral rehydration solution designed specifically for children and infants.

- Do not give over-the-counter antidiarrheal medications to children younger than 2 years. In older children, use these medications under the guidance of a healthcare provider.

When a child has vomiting, diarrhea or both, consult a healthcare provider if:

- The diarrhea or vomiting persists for more than a few days.

- The child or infant is not able to keep fluids down.

- The child or infant has not had a wet diaper in 3 or more hours (or, if toilet-trained, has not urinated for more than 6 hours).

- The child has a high fever.

- The diarrhea is bloody or black.

- The child is unusually sleepy or irritable.

- The child cries without tears or has a dry mouth.

- There is a sunken appearance to the child's abdomen, eyes or cheeks (or, in a very young infant, the soft spot at the top of the infant's head).

- The child's skin remains "tented" if pinched and released.

# Respiratory Distress

For children, respiratory distress is the second-most common emergency condition. Children are more susceptible than adults to respiratory distress because their airways are smaller, narrower and less rigid. In addition to the signs and symptoms of respiratory distress seen in adults (see Chapter 5), children may have the following signs and symptoms:

- Nasal flaring (widening of the nostrils when breathing in)

- Use of the chest and neck muscles to breathe (muscles pull in around the collarbone and ribs)

- Grunting

Two common infections associated with respiratory distress in children are croup and epiglottitis.

- **Croup (laryngotracheobronchitis)** is an infection of the upper airway that causes difficulty breathing and a harsh, repetitive, bark-like cough. When the child breathes in, he or she may make a high-pitched whistling noise. Croup is most common in children younger than 5 years. Croup usually is not serious and can be managed at home; however, in some cases, a child with croup can progress quickly from respiratory distress to respiratory arrest.

- **Epiglottitis** is swelling of the epiglottis (the piece of cartilage that covers the trachea), usually caused by a bacterial infection. Epiglottitis is life threatening because the swelling can block the windpipe and lead to severe breathing problems. Since the implementation of routine vaccination against *H. influenza* type B with the Hib vaccine, the number of cases of epiglottitis has dropped significantly in the United States.

## General Strategies for Reducing the Risk for Injury

- Think and act with safety in mind.

- Be aware of your environment and surroundings.

- Dress appropriately for the weather and your planned activity.

- Read and follow instructions and safety guidelines.

- Use safety equipment that is available to you (e.g., seat belts, helmets, protective eyewear and footwear).

- Get trained in first aid, CPR and AED use, and keep your knowledge and skills current. To enroll in a Red Cross first aid/CPR/AED class, visit redcross.org.

- Have an emergency action plan (Box D-1).

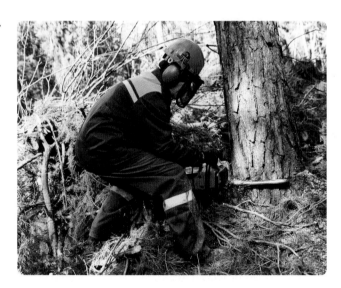

## Box D-1. **Developing an Emergency Action Plan**

Emergencies happen quickly. There may not be time to consider what to do, only time to react. Having an emergency action plan in place and being familiar with the procedures it contains can save precious minutes when every minute counts. To create an emergency action plan:

1. Identify the types of emergencies that could occur. Think about potential injuries, illnesses, weather events and other situations (such as power failures) that are likely to occur in your specific setting.

2. Develop and write down the procedure that is to be followed in the event of each emergency. Include:

   - The signal that will be used to indicate that the emergency action plan should be activated (such as a whistle blast).

   - The steps for responding to the emergency, and who is responsible for each step.

   - The procedure for calling 9-1-1 or the designated emergency number and directing emergency medical services (EMS) personnel to the scene.

   - What follow-up actions should be taken, if any.

3. Identify equipment that is needed to respond to the potential emergencies you have identified and stock it in an easily accessible place.

Review the emergency action plan with family members, and practice it regularly so that the procedures it contains become second nature. Periodically review the emergency action plan and update it as necessary.

# Vehicle Safety

- Do not use alcohol or drugs while operating a motor vehicle.

- Do not drive distracted. Texting, emailing or talking on a mobile phone; eating or drinking; talking to passengers; reading; using navigation systems; operating audiovisual equipment; daydreaming; and putting on makeup are hazardous activities when you are behind the wheel.

- Do not drive drowsy. Lack of sleep affects your ability to operate a vehicle safely, even if you do not actually fall asleep at the wheel. When you are not well rested, your reaction time is slowed and your judgment is impaired. Know the warning signs that you are too tired to drive: yawning or blinking frequently, drifting from your lane, missing an exit or not being able to recall driving for the last several miles. Pull over to rest or change drivers. Opening the window for fresh air or drinking a caffeinated beverage will not keep you alert enough to continue driving.

- Always wear your seat belt.

- Always have infants and children younger than 12 years ride in the back seat in safety seats that are approved for the child's age and size (Figure D-1). The amount of force created by a deploying airbag can kill or severely injure an infant or child occupying the front seat, even if the infant or child is in a rear-facing safety seat. Make sure that the safety seat is installed correctly in your vehicle. Visit the National Highway Traffic Safety Administration website (nhtsa.gov) for information about choosing an appropriate child safety seat and using it correctly. If you need help installing the safety seat or want to be sure that you have installed the seat correctly, visit safecar.gov to find a nearby child safety seat inspection station.

- Never leave a child alone in a car, even for a few minutes, and always check the backseat of the vehicle before you lock it and walk away. Temperatures inside the car can reach deadly levels quickly, even when the temperature outside is moderate.

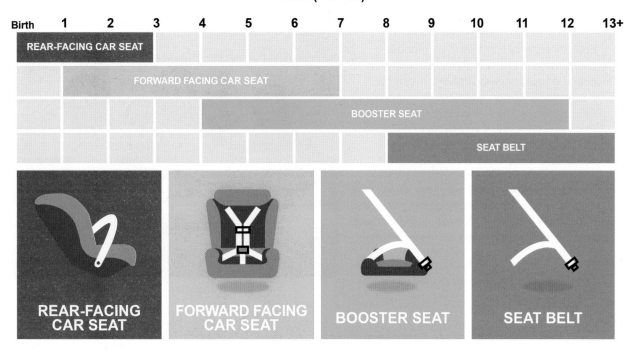

| | Birth | 1 | 2 | 3 | 4 | 5 | 6 | 7 | 8 | 9 | 10 | 11 | 12 | 13+ |
|---|---|---|---|---|---|---|---|---|---|---|---|---|---|---|
| REAR-FACING CAR SEAT | | | | | | | | | | | | | | |
| FORWARD FACING CAR SEAT | | | | | | | | | | | | | | |
| BOOSTER SEAT | | | | | | | | | | | | | | |
| SEAT BELT | | | | | | | | | | | | | | |

**REAR-FACING CAR SEAT** **FORWARD FACING CAR SEAT** **BOOSTER SEAT** **SEAT BELT**

**Figure D-1.** The National Highway Traffic Safety Administration provides car seat recommendations for children from birth through 12 years.

# Fire Safety

- Install a smoke alarm and carbon monoxide detector on every floor of your home. Check the batteries once a month, and change the batteries at least every 6 months.

- Make sure that your home has at least one working, easily accessible fire extinguisher, and make sure everyone in your home knows how to use it.

- Have fireplaces and chimneys inspected annually and perform cleaning and repairs as necessary.

- Develop and practice a fire escape plan with your family. Gather everyone together at a convenient time. For each floor of your home, sketch a floor plan, noting rooms, doors, windows and hallways. Use arrows to indicate two ways (if possible) to get out of each room. Teach family members to leave the building first, then call 9-1-1 or the designated emergency number. No one should re-enter the burning building for any reason. To escape:

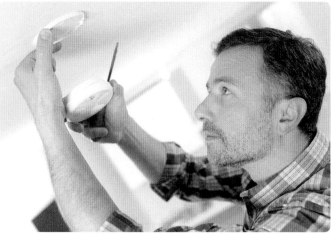

- Feel the door first. Do not open it if it is hot.

- If smoke is present, crawl low.

- If escape is not possible, stay in the room and call 9-1-1 or the designated emergency number, even if rescuers are already outside.

# Safety at Home

- Enter emergency numbers in your mobile phone's contact list and post them near every phone in your home. Include 9-1-1 or the designated emergency number, the national Poison Help hotline (1-800-222-1222), and the phone numbers of your family's healthcare providers, as well as any other important numbers.

- Make an emergency preparedness kit and have an emergency preparedness plan in place. Visit redcross.org for more information about how to prepare for disasters and other emergencies.

- Box D-2 contains a checklist of special safety considerations for households with young children.

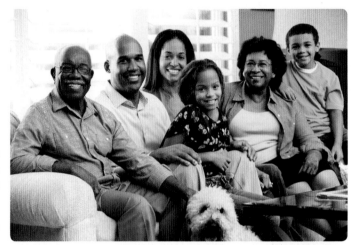

## Box D-2. **A Safety Checklist for Households with Young Children**

### To Prevent Fire and Burns

☐ Matches and lighters are stored out of the reach of children.

☐ Space heaters, if used, are placed out of the reach of children and away from curtains.

☐ Pot and pan handles are turned toward the back of the stove and out of the reach of children.

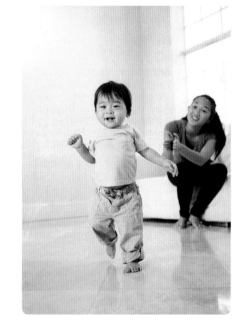

### To Prevent Electrical Shock

☐ Safety covers are placed on all unused electrical outlets.

☐ Loose cords are secured and out of the way.

☐ Electrical appliances are away from sinks, tubs, toilets and other sources of water.

### To Prevent Choking, Suffocation and Strangulation

☐ Small objects are kept out of children's reach.

☐ Toys are age appropriate and pose no choking hazard.

☐ Items such as coolers and plastic storage containers that a child could get trapped in are stored in a safe place that is not accessible to the child.

*(Continued)*

- [ ] Lidded toy boxes have lightweight, removable lids with supports to keep the lids open and air vents to allow air flow when the lid is closed.

- [ ] The crib mattress fits into the crib snugly, and all soft objects and loose bedding (such as toys, blankets, bumper pads and pillows) are removed from the crib. The only thing in the crib is a mattress with a tightly fitting sheet.

## To Prevent Drowning

- [ ] Swimming pools and hot tubs are completely surrounded with a fence, and the gate to the fence is locked. Hot tubs are covered, and the cover is secured.

- [ ] Kiddie pools, bathtubs and sinks are immediately emptied after each use.

- [ ] Toilet lids are kept down when not in use.

## To Prevent Poisoning

- [ ] Cleaning supplies, laundry supplies, car maintenance supplies, pesticides and other household chemicals are stored in locked cabinets and are out of the reach of children.

- [ ] Houseplants are kept out of reach.

## To Prevent Falls and Tipping Injuries

- [ ] Safety gates are installed at all open stairways in homes with toddlers and babies. (Note: Pressure gates, which attach to the walls with pressure rather than with screws, should not be installed at the top of stairs. This type of gate can give way if a child leans on it.)

- [ ] Windows and balcony doors have childproof latches or window guards.

## To Prevent Wounds

- [ ] Knives, hand tools, power tools, razor blades, scissors, guns, ammunition and other objects that can cause injury are stored in locked cabinets or locked storage areas.

- [ ] Drape and blind cords are wound up and not dangling.

- [ ] Objects with cords, strings or ribbons are kept out of the reach of children. Hanging crib toys, like mobiles, are removed from cribs when the baby first begins to push up on his or her hands and knees or when the baby is 5 months old, whichever occurs first.

- [ ] Bathroom and laundry room doors are kept closed at all times.

- [ ] Buckets or other containers with standing water are securely covered or emptied of water and stored upside-down and out of children's reach.

- [ ] Medicine is kept in a locked storage place that children cannot reach.

- [ ] Packages containing potential poisons are closed securely after each use, and the container is promptly returned to a locked cabinet. (Note: There is no such thing as "childproof" packaging.)

- [ ] Balconies have barriers to prevent children from slipping through the bars.

- [ ] Large, heavy items (such as television sets, microwaves, fish tanks, dressers, bookcases and heavy appliances) are properly secured to the wall to prevent them from tipping over onto a child if the child climbs or hangs on them.

- [ ] Corner guards are installed on all sharp furniture edges.

# Preventing Slips, Trips and Falls

- Make sure that stairways and hallways are well lit.

- Make sure that stairways and hallways are free of clutter.

- Equip stairways with handrails, and use nonslip treads or securely fastened rugs.

- Secure rugs to the floor with double-sided tape.

- Ensure that cords for lamps and other items are not placed where someone can trip over them.

- Clean up spills promptly.

- Place a mat with a suction base of the bottom of the tub if the tub does not have built-in nonslip strips.

- If a member of your household has impaired mobility, install handrails in the bathtub or shower and beside the toilet.

# Preventing Burns and Fires

- Set the water heater at a temperature of 120° F or less to prevent scalding. If your household contains children or older adults, the water temperature should be lower, between 100° F and 115° F.

- Keep flammable items, such as curtains, away from heat sources, such as space heaters.

- Do not wear loose clothing when cooking.

- When you are using the stove, use the back burners and turn pot and pan handles toward the back of the stove so that they are out of the reach of children.

- Do not use extension cords or overload outlets.

# Preventing Firearm Accidents

- Keep firearms in the home unloaded in a locked place, out of the reach of children. Store ammunition separately in a locked location.

- Obtain the knowledge and skills you need to handle firearms safely.

# Safety at Work

At work, participate in any workplace safety programs your employer offers. Make sure you know:

- Your place of employment's emergency action plan and fire evacuation procedures.

- How to activate your emergency response team and how to call 9-1-1 or the designated emergency number.

- The location of the nearest fire extinguisher, automated external defibrillator (AED) and first aid kit.

- How to use recommended safety equipment and how to follow safety procedures if you work in an environment where hazards exist.

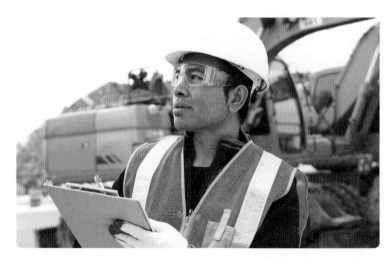

# Safety at Play

Enjoy sports and other recreational activities safely by making sure equipment is in good working order and following accepted guidelines for the activity. Before undertaking an activity that is unfamiliar to you, such as boating, skiing or riding a motorcycle, take lessons to learn how to perform the activity safely.

## Water Safety

- Learn to swim and obtain the knowledge and skills you need to prevent, recognize and respond to aquatic emergencies. Knowing how to swim is a basic life skill that everyone should possess. The American Red Cross Swimming and Water Safety program teaches people to be safe in, on and around the water through water safety courses, water orientation classes for infants and toddlers, and comprehensive Learn-to-Swim courses for people of all ages and abilities.

- Use a U.S. Coast Guard–approved life jacket. Young children, weak or inexperienced swimmers and nonswimmers should always wear a U.S. Coast Guard–approved life jacket whenever they are in, on or around the water. Even strong swimmers should wear a U.S. Coast Guard–approved life jacket when engaging in certain aquatic activities, such as boating.

- Do not use alcohol or drugs while engaging in aquatic activities.

- Never swim alone. Swim only in designated areas and areas supervised by a lifeguard.

- Closely supervise children in, on or near water, even when a lifeguard is present. Stay within arm's reach of the child.

- Read and obey all rules and posted signs. Pay special attention to water-depth markings and "no diving" signs.

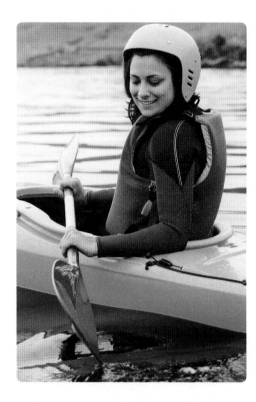

- Enter the water feetfirst, unless you are in an area that is clearly marked for diving and has no obstructions.

- Watch out for the dangerous "too's": too tired, too cold, too far away from safety, too much sun and too much strenuous activity.

# Bicycle Safety

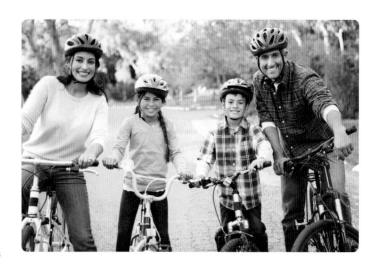

- Always wear an approved helmet. Children should wear a helmet even if they are still riding along the sidewalk on training wheels. Look for a helmet that has been approved by the Snell Memorial Foundation or the American National Standards Institute (ANSI), and make that sure the helmet is the correct size and that it fits comfortably and securely. Laws on wearing bicycle helmets, including age-specific requirements, vary by state and county. For more information about helmet laws in your area, conduct an Internet search or contact state or local officials.

- Avoid riding on roads that are busy or have no shoulder.

- Wear reflective clothing at night.

- Use a headlight, taillight and high-visibility strobe lights on your bicycle wheels.

- Keep bicycles properly maintained.

# Safety for Runners, Joggers and Walkers

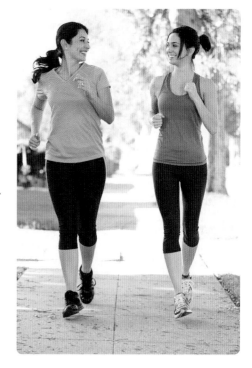

- Plan your route carefully and exercise in well-lit, well-populated areas.

- Consider exercising with another person.

- Pay attention to your environment and surroundings. Consider exercising without music.

- Avoid roads that do not easily accommodate pedestrian traffic.

- If you must exercise outdoors after dark, wear reflective clothing and run, jog or walk facing traffic.

- Be alert for cars pulling out at intersections and driveways.

# GLOSSARY

## A

**Abdominal thrusts:** inward and upward thrusts just above the navel, used in combination with back blows to force the object out of the airway when a person is choking

**Abrasion:** an open wound that occurs when something rubs roughly against the skin, causing damage to the skin's surface

**Abuse:** the willful infliction of injury or harm on another

**Acute illness:** an illness that strikes suddenly and usually only lasts for a short period of time

**Agonal breaths:** isolated or infrequent gasping in the absence of normal breathing in an unresponsive person

**Airborne pathogens:** disease-causing micro-organisms that are expelled into the air when an infected person breathes, coughs or sneezes

**Anaphylaxis:** a severe, life-threatening allergic reaction

**Antihistamine:** a medication that counteracts the effects of histamine, a chemical released by the body during an allergic reaction

**Asthma:** a chronic illness in which certain substances or conditions (triggers) cause inflammation and narrowing of the airways, making breathing difficult

**Asthma action plan:** a written plan that the person develops with his or her healthcare provider that details daily management of the condition as well as how to handle an asthma attack

**Aura:** an unusual sensation or feeling that may signal the onset of a seizure in some people

**Avulsion:** an open wound that occurs when a portion of the skin, and sometimes the underlying tissue, is partially or completely torn away

## B

**Back blows:** blows between the shoulder blades, used in combination with abdominal thrusts to force the object out of the airway when a person is choking

**Bandage:** a strip of material used to hold a dressing in place and to control bleeding

**Bloodborne pathogens:** disease-causing microorganisms that are spread when blood from an infected person enters the bloodstream of a person who is not infected

**Blunt trauma:** injury caused by impact with a flat object or surface

**Brain contusion:** bruising of the brain tissue

**Brain hematoma:** bleeding into the space between the brain and the skull

**Breathing barriers:** devices used to protect the responder from contact with saliva and other body fluids, such as blood, when giving rescue breaths

**Bruise:** a type of closed wound that occurs when the small blood vessels under the surface of the skin are damaged and blood leaks into the surrounding tissues

**Burn:** a traumatic injury to the skin (and sometimes the underlying tissues as well) caused by contact with extreme heat, chemicals, radiation or electricity

## C

**Cardiac arrest:** a condition that occurs when the heart stops beating or beats too ineffectively to circulate blood to the brain and other vital organs

**Cardiac Chain of Survival:** five actions that, when performed in rapid succession, increase a person's likelihood of surviving cardiac arrest

**Chronic illness:** an illness that a person lives with on an ongoing basis and that often requires continuous treatment to manage

**Closed wound:** a wound where the surface of the skin is intact but the underlying tissues are injured

**Compression-only CPR:** a CPR technique that involves giving continuous chest compressions, with no rescue breaths

**Concussion:** a traumatic brain injury that alters the way the brain functions

**Consent:** permission to give care

**Convulsions:** uncontrolled body movements caused by contraction of the muscles

**CPR:** cardiopulmonary resuscitation; a skill that is used when a person is in cardiac arrest to keep oxygenated blood moving to the brain and other vital organs until advanced medical help arrives

**Croup (laryngotracheobronchitis):** an infection of the upper airway that causes difficulty breathing and a harsh, repetitive, bark-like cough; common in children younger than 5 years

# D

**Dehydration:** too little fluid in the body

**Diabetes:** a chronic condition characterized by the body's inability to process glucose (sugar) in the bloodstream

**Diffuse axonal injury:** tearing of nerves throughout the brain tissue

**Dislocation:** an injury that occurs when the bones that meet at a joint move out of their normal position

**Dressing:** a pad that is placed directly on a wound to absorb blood and other fluids, promote clotting and prevent infection

# E

**Emergency medical services (EMS) system:** a network of professionals linked together to provide the best care for people in all types of emergencies

**Epiglottitis:** swelling of the epiglottis (the piece of cartilage that covers the trachea), usually caused by a bacterial infection

**Epilepsy:** a chronic seizure disorder that can often be controlled with medication

**Epinephrine:** a drug that slows or stops the effects of anaphylaxis

**Epinephrine auto injector:** a syringe system, available by prescription only, that contains a single dose of epinephrine

**External bleeding:** bleeding that is visible on the outside of the body

# F

**Face shield:** a breathing barrier used to protect the responder from contact with saliva and other body fluids, such as blood, as he or she gives rescue breaths; consists of a flat piece of thin plastic that is placed over the person's face with the opening over the person's mouth

**Febrile seizure:** a convulsion brought on by a fever in an infant or small child

**Fracture:** a complete break, a chip or a crack in a bone

**Frostbite:** an injury caused by freezing of the skin and underlying tissues as a result of prolonged exposure to freezing or subfreezing temperatures

# G

**Good Samaritan laws:** laws that protect people against claims of negligence when they give emergency care in good faith without accepting anything in return

# H

**Head-tilt/chin-lift maneuver:** a technique used to open the airway

**Heart attack:** a condition that occurs when blood flow to part of the heart muscle is blocked (e.g., as a result of coronary artery disease), causing cells in the affected area of the heart muscle to die

**Heat cramps:** painful muscle spasms, usually in the legs and abdomen, caused by loss of fluids and electrolytes as a result of sweating

**Heat exhaustion:** a condition that occurs when fluids lost through sweating are not replaced

**Heat stroke:** a life-threatening condition that occurs when the body's cooling system is completely overwhelmed and stops working

**Hemostatic dressing:** a dressing treated with a substance that speeds clot formation

**Hyperglycemia:** excessively high blood glucose levels

**Hyperventilation:** breathing that is faster and shallower than normal

**Hypoglycemia:** excessively low blood glucose levels

**Hypothermia:** a condition that occurs when the body loses heat faster than it can produce heat, causing the core body temperature to fall below 95° F (35° C)

## I

**Implied consent:** permission to give care that is not expressly granted by the person but is assumed because circumstances exist that would lead a reasonable person to believe that the person would give consent if he or she were able to

**Insulin:** a hormone secreted by the pancreas that causes glucose to be moved from the bloodstream into the cells, where it is used for energy

**Internal bleeding:** bleeding that occurs inside the body, into a body cavity or space

## L

**Laceration:** a cut, commonly caused by a sharp object such as broken glass or a knife

**Lay responder:** a nonprofessional responder who gives care in an emergency situation

**Long-term control medications:** medications taken regularly to help prevent asthma attacks by reducing inflammation and swelling and making the airways less sensitive to triggers

**Lung contusion:** bruising of the lung tissue

## O

**Open wound:** a wound where the skin's surface is broken

## P

**Paradoxical breathing:** abnormal movement of the chest wall when a person breathes (when the person inhales, the injured area draws in while the rest of the chest expands and when the person exhales, the injured area expands while the rest of the chest draws in)

**Paralysis:** the loss of movement, sensation or both

**Paraplegia:** paralysis that affects both legs and the lower trunk

**Pathogens:** harmful microorganisms that can cause disease

**Penetrating trauma:** trauma that occurs when the body is pierced by or impaled on a sharp, narrow object

**Personal protective equipment (PPE):** barrier devices used to prevent pathogens from contaminating the skin, mucous membranes or clothing

**Pneumothorax:** collapse of a lung caused by an abnormal collection of air in the space between the lung and the chest wall

**Pocket mask:** a transparent, flexible device that creates a tight seal over the person's nose and mouth to allow the responder to give rescue breaths without making mouth-to-mouth contact or inhaling exhaled air; a type of breathing barrier

**Puncture wound:** an open wound that occurs when a pointed object, such as a nail or an animal's tooth, pierces the skin

## Q

**Quadriplegia:** paralysis that affects both arms, the trunk and both legs

**Quick-relief (rescue) medications:** medications taken when a person is experiencing an acute asthma attack to open the airways right away

## R

**Respiratory arrest:** absence of breathing

**Respiratory distress:** difficulty breathing

## S

**Scene size-up:** a brief survey done prior to entering the scene of an emergency to ensure safety, form an initial impression about what happened and the nature of the person's illness or injury, identify any life-threatening conditions, and determine necessary resources

**Seizure:** a temporary and involuntary change in body movement, function, sensation, awareness or behavior that results from abnormal electrical activity in the brain

**Shock:** a progressive, life-threatening condition in which the circulatory system fails to deliver enough oxygen-rich blood to the body's tissues and organs, causing organs and body systems to begin to fail

**Sprain:** an injury that occurs when a ligament is stretched, torn or damaged (ligaments connect bones to bones at the joints)

**Strain:** an injury that occurs when a tendon or muscle is stretched, torn or damaged (tendons connect muscles to bones)

**Stroke:** a condition that occurs when blood flow to part of the brain is interrupted by a blood clot, causing cells in the affected area of the brain to die; can also result from bleeding into the brain tissue

**Sudden cardiac arrest:** cardiac arrest that happens suddenly and without any warning signs

# T

**Tetanus:** a severe bacterial infection that can result from a puncture wound or a deep laceration

**Thermoregulation:** the body's ability to maintain an internal temperature within an acceptable range despite external conditions

**Tourniquet:** a device placed around an arm or leg to constrict blood vessels and stop blood flow to a wound

**Tracheostomy:** a surgically created opening in the front of the neck that opens into the trachea (windpipe) to form an alternate route for breathing when the upper airway is blocked or damaged

**Transient ischemic attack (TIA):** a condition that occurs when blood flow to part of the brain is temporarily interrupted, causing stroke-like signs and symptoms that then go away

**Triggers:** substances or conditions that initiate an asthma attack when the person is exposed to them

# U

**Urushiol:** an oil on plants such as poison ivy, poison sumac and poison oak that causes an allergic skin reaction in many people

# V

**Ventricular fibrillation (V-fib):** an abnormal heart rhythm in which the heart muscle simply quivers (fibrillates) weakly instead of contracting strongly

**Ventricular tachycardia (V-tach):** an abnormal heart rhythm in which the heart muscle contracts too fast

# W

**Wound:** an injury that results when the skin or other tissues of the body are damaged

# SOURCES

American Academy of Allergy, Asthma and Immunology. *Food Allergy.* http://www.aaaai.org /patients/gallery/foodallergy.asp. Accessed October 2015.

American Diabetes Association. *Living with Diabetes: Hyperglycemia (High Blood Glucose).* http://www .diabetes.org/living-with-diabetes/treatment-and-care/blood-glucose-control/hyperglycemia.html. Accessed October 2015.

American Diabetes Association. *Living with Diabetes: Hypoglycemia (Low Blood Glucose).* http://www .diabetes.org/living-with-diabetes/treatment-and-care/blood-glucose-control/hypoglycemia-low-blood.html. Accessed October 2015.

American Heart Association. *CPR Facts and Stats.* http://cpr.heart.org/AHAECC/CPRAndECC/ AboutCPRFirstAid/CPRFactsAndStats/UCM_475748_CPR-Facts-and-Stats.jsp. Accessed October 2015.

American Lung Association. *Asthma.* http://www.lung.org/lung-health-and-diseases/lung-disease-lookup /asthma/. Accessed October 2015.

Asthma and Allergy Foundation of America: *Asthma Overview.* http://www.aafa.org/display .cfm?id=8&cont=8. Accessed October 2015.

Centers for Disease Control and Prevention. *Prevent Lyme Disease.* http://www.cdc.gov/Features/ LymeDisease/. Accessed October 2015.

Home Safety Council. *Safety Tips: Poison.* http://homesafetycouncil.org/SafetyGuide/sg_poison_w001.asp. Accessed September 2015.

MayoClinic.com. *Hypothermia: Risk Factors.* http://www.mayoclinic.org/diseases-conditions/hypothermia/ basics/risk-factors/CON-20020453. Accessed October 2015.

MedlinePlus. *Epiglottitis.* https://www.nlm.nih.gov/medlineplus/ency/article/000605.htm. Accessed October 2015.

MedlinePlus. *Hypothermia.* http://www.nlm.nih.gov/medlineplus/hypothermia.html. Accessed October 2015.

National Highway Traffic Safety Administration. *Car Seat By Child's Age and Size.* http://www.safercar.gov/ parents/CarSeats/Right-Car-Seat-Age-Size.htm. Accessed October 2015.

REI. *Layering Basics.* http://www.rei.com/expertadvice/articles/dress+layers.html. Accessed October 2015.

Title 42 United States Code Section 1395 cc (a)(1)(Q)(A).Patient Self-Determination Act.

United States Department of Health and Human Services. *The Poison Help Line.* http://poisonhelp.hrsa.gov/ the-poison-help-line/index.html. Accessed October 2015.

United States Department of Justice. *Burn Injuries in Child Abuse.* https://www.ncjrs.gov/pdffiles/91190-6 .pdf. Accessed October 2015.

United States Department of Labor. *Welcome to OSHA's Campaign to Prevent Heat Illness in Outdoor Workers.* https://www.osha.gov/SLTC/heatillness/index.html. Accessed October 2015.

United States Federal Communications Commission. *Guide: 911 Wireless Services.* https://www.fcc.gov /guides/wireless-911-services. Accessed October 2015.

United States National Library of Medicine. *Transient Ischemic Attack.* http://www.nlm.nih.gov/medlineplus /ency/article/000730.htm. Accessed October 2015.

# PHOTOGRAPHY CREDITS

## Chapter 1

Page

4    Photo by N-StyleID.com

6    iStock.com/Daniel Stein

9    D. Hammonds/Shutterstock.com

10   iStock.com/katifcam

14   Gang Liu/Shutterstock.com

16   MegaPixel/Shutterstock.com

## Chapter 3

Page

36   Ronald Sumners/Shutterstock.com

37   Leigh Prather/Shutterstock.com

42   Courtesy of Zoll Medical Corporation

48   Courtesy of Zoll Medical Corporation

49   Paul Velgos/Shutterstock.com

## Chapter 4

Page

62   © iStock.com/NakedRhino

62   © iStock.com/Ekely

## Chapter 5

Page

76   iStock.com/Izabela Habur

76   Photo by N-StyleID.com

78   Peter Bernik/Shutterstock.com

79   Bayanova Svetlana/Shutterstock.com

79   iStock.com/davidf

79   iStock.com/saritwuttisan

79   iStock.com/flubydust

80   iStock.com/jjpoole

82   EpiPen® is a registered trademark owned by the Mylan companies.

## Chapter 6

Page

97    Kondor83/Shutterstock.com

97    iStock.com/conmesa

97    iStock.com/conmesa

97    sima/Shutterstock.com

98    Winai Tepsuttinun/Shutterstock.com

98    Zerzaaman/Shutterstock.com

99    rangizzz/Shutterstock.com

100   Picsfive/Shutterstock.com

100   design56/Shutterstock.com

102   Courtesy of Tactical Medical Solutions, Inc.

105   Marcin Balcerzak/Shutterstock.com

106   michaeljung/Shutterstock.com

109   iStock.com/robeo

110   SergiyN/Shutterstock.com

111   iStock.com/monkeybusinessimages

## Chapter 7

Page

118   iStock.com/ilkercelik

119   VR Photos/Shutterstock.com

121   Filaphoto/Shutterstock.com

121   iStock.com/skibrek

124   Juliya_strekoza/Shutterstock.com

## Appendix D

# INDEX

Note: *b* indicates box; *f*, figure; and *t*, table.

pelvic, 115
  shock and, 94
Triangular bandage, 108, 108*f*
Trigger, 78
Trip prevention, 153*b,* 154
Tuberculosis, 12*b*
Two-person seat carry, 142

Unresponsive person
  checking of, 28–29, 32–33
  description of, 18
  following choking, 67, 69, 71, 73
Urushiol oil, 136

Vehicle safety, 150, 151*f*
Venomous snakes, 130*t*

Venomous spiders, 132*t*
Ventricular fibrillation (V-fib), 42
Ventricular tachycardia (V-tach), 42
Vomiting, in children, 147

Wading assist, 17*b*
Walking assist, 141
Walking safety, 156
Water moccasin (cottonmouth) snake, 130*t*
Water safety, 155
Work safety, 154
Wounds
  children and prevention of, 153*b*
  closed, 95–96
  open, 96–103 (*See also* open wound[s])
  treating infection in, 99*b*